# Xcel Wellness Tai Chi

J Pilgrim

Published by Xcel Wellness, 2024.

While every precaution has been taken in the preparation of this book, the publisher assumes no responsibility for errors or omissions, or for damages resulting from the use of the information contained herein.

XCEL WELLNESS TAI CHI

**First edition. February 17, 2024.**



ISBN: 979-8224402144

Written by J Pilgrim.

# Also by J Pilgrim

**The Trionian Saga**
The Trionian Saga - Part One: Beyond the Border Mountains
The Trionian Saga - Part Two: The Hyna Sword
The Trionian Saga - Part Three: The Quest for Lyla

**Standalone**
The Hens in Poultsville
Sleeping with Crystal
Excel Your Wellness: Virtues and Vitamins
The Chi Key: Reflections on You, Me, and the Universe
Body Strengthening Strategy
Xcel Wellness Tai Chi

Watch for more at www.thetrioniansaga.weebly.com.

# Table of Contents

# Xcelwellness Tai Chi Program

Xcelwellness Tai Chi takes a holistic approach to health and well-being with each session involving gentle stretching, relaxation, energization, and total body balancing treatments. This 'feel good' therapy enhances one's overall health status for life, work, and play. Xcelwellness Tai Chi can help if you suffer from general poor health, stiffness, and fatigue.

XCELWELLNESS TAI CHI FOR BUSY PEOPLE IN YOUR OWN TIME, OWN PACE AND OWN PLACE!

Use Xcelwellness Tai Chi to prepare for the workday, to be more focused on activities, to energize, and to sleep more deeply. The comprehensive fitness program with step-by-step guidance for any age group, any place, to fit any lifestyle and schedule.

Tai Chi has been referred to as Yoga in Motion, a moving meditation and a stand-up massage - a powerful key to relaxation, increased focus, and well-being. Xcelwellness Tai Chi can make a big difference for healthy, but very busy people - here is how:

- Improve Flexibility for Sports People

- **Help Recovery after an Illness**

- Provide Exercise for the Disabled

- **Reduce Stress and Improve Energy Levels**

<u>Xcelwellness Tai Chi</u>

The Tai Chi Form presented in this book is a short version of the Cheng Man Ching style (and the popular Yang style).

<u>Tai Chi has its ancient alliances in two internal art forms:</u>

<u>Martial Arts:</u> Tai Chi is an ancient elite Chinese martial art. Postures are martial art stances. The practitioner can explore the defensive and attacking aspects during practice.

<u>Chi Kung (Qigong):</u> This art is the basis behind martial arts as it is interested in generating internal Chi power by holding postures for longer while directing the breath and meditating on the flow of life force around the meridians and chakra vortexes. In advanced Tai Chi practice, one has the option of holding the postures for longer periods and working with the energy flow in the body.

In the Form, there are three sections - with five posture-sets in each section. Some of the posture-sets are repeated in the Form.

The posture sets are demonstrated through images with explanations of each move encouraging physical participation. The book covers breathing re-training, stances, and relaxation techniques and features remarkable posture-sets such as: Grasping Sparrows Tail, Diagonal Flying, Fair Lady Weaves the Shuttle, Wave Hands in Clouds, and Shoulder Stroke.

The entire Form takes the participant around in a circle embracing the poles of North, East, South, and West. The directions to face and move, which are explained in the text, give the participant a reference to work from.

The floor space required to perform the entire Tai Chi Form is no more than a three-metre span squared.

## Section One: Ease and Relax

Focusing on nurturing inner harmony in one's life, these Five Posture-Sets are demonstrated with an explanation of each move. Your participation in Xcelwellness Tai Chi has the potential to:

- Relax the Musculature aiding Circulation

- Help Overcome When Overwhelmed

- Enhance Inner Harmony

- Boost Confidence


## Section Two: Cleanse and Instil

Focusing on an inner spring-clean in one's life, these Five Posture-Sets are demonstrated with an explanation of each move. Your participation in Xcelwellness Tai Chi has the potential to:

- Clear Mental Clutter improving Thought Processes

- Balance the Secretion of Hormones and Purify the Body

- Help get Retained Emotions off the Chest


## Section Three: Energize and Empower

Focusing on enhancing Chi power in one's life, these Five Posture-Sets are demonstrated with an explanation of each move. Your participation in Xcelwellness Tai Chi has the potential to:

- Revitalize body and mind with Renewed Energy and Zest for Life

- Enhance Natural Cycles and Functioning of all Bodily Systems

- Increase Flexibility for overall Well-being

## <u>Welcome to this Course</u>

Mirroring real natural life, Tai Chi postures begin, change, and end, only to be reborn to repeat the cycle on the other side of the body. The practitioner keeps this in mind while moving the body, arms, and legs from one posture to the next, helping transitions to be smooth and controlled.

First, to achieve central equilibrium, one can imagine a white light entering through the crown cascading down through the body, and exiting into the earth. This then splits the body into two sides: left and right. Both sides represent the cycle of birth, growth, conclusion, and rebirth. For example, the left side is heavy and closed while the right side is light and open - and then during the next posture, the left side is light and open, while the right side is heavy and closed - always evolving.

The beginner learns the mechanics of the posture sets first, but as confidence builds the focus turns to moving from one's center (initiating moves from the core just below the navel) which assists in smooth silk-like moves and the generation of Chi power and energy flow.

During the session, the participant can explore different aspects such as breathing or grounding; peripheral vision or senses; lightness or heaviness; open or closed; fast or slow; full or empty; and hard or soft. These qualities add further dimensions to practice. This keeps regular practice interesting, and concentration on these aspects flows into everyday life, aiding one to be more aware and focused at home, work, and play.

<u>Incorrect posture</u> impairs core strength, escalating muscular fatigue and stiffness to the legs, shoulders, back, and neck. Further, these areas become inflamed and aggravated by repetitious activity in a day.

Such imbalances can be corrected by <u>Xcelwellness Tai Chi</u> which counters dysfunctional muscle activity by:

- Applying gentle stretches, muscle tension is eased

- **Pelvic tilt is corrected to restore proper body position**

- Trigger points in muscles are addressed to relieve overload

- **Circulation and energy flow is restored to the muscle groups**

- A full body workout with all meridian lines stretched and acupressure points activated.

With any exercise program, one should be careful and ease into the form gradually. It is best practice to follow the outline in this book to warm up adequately before undertaking the workout, and then to perform the cool-down exercises to finish. Remember to hydrate and take in protein to aid muscle development.

Remember to practice deep slow breathing during the form, timing the breathing with the stretch. Deep diaphragm breathing benefits cellular health, calms the nervous system, and increases lung capacity.

Before you do the entire series of movements from beginning to end which usually takes ten minutes for the accomplished practitioner, allow your mind to put aside the concerns of this world. Put on some soothing music, and get ready for a powerful liberating experience with Xcelwellness Tai Chi.

Tai Chi is a healing art and works on all levels of health and well-being, with the potential to downscale degenerative diseases and promote longevity. Xcelwellness Tai Chi can increase the flexibility of your joints, massage internal organs, and benefit circulation.

Tai Chi is a holistic practice, that benefits the mind and emotions, improving concentration, awareness, outlook, and vitality.

*"With regular daily practice, I have noticed results in the form of a constant energy supply and a detoxification of my system. I feel an all-round feeling of goodness and solidarity in my body. I am sleeping more soundly and enjoy a more pain-free life." John T, 45 yrs.*

*"Hi, I love your tai chi - so clear & concise and easy to follow with step-by-step guidance. I am telling my friends about the course too, thanks xcelwellness!" Jean P, 31 yrs.*

*"I was ailing in health and needed a pick-me-up. Your tai chi course has helped me get my health back on track. I practice daily and feel the energy and vitality in my body. The sore spots have vanished and when I feel stiff, just ten minutes of tai chi gets my circulation going again." Thomas G, 62 yrs.*

*"I've been looking for a tai chi course like yours for ages with an easy simple explanation and a short form that takes a few minutes to complete. I feel the benefits immediately after each run-through and I'll proceed with the next section shortly. Thanks." Gordon W, 23 yrs.*

### *Practice These Bonus Positive Affirmations During The Session To Re-Train The Mind*

*- I AM VIBRANT AND ALIVE*

*- **I AM HAPPY AND HEALTHY***

*- I AM CALM AND CONFIDENT*

*- **I AM WISE AND SUCCESSFUL***

*- I AM YOUNG AND STRONG*

People who allow Tai Chi to be a part of their life, experience a removal of debilitating mental blocks, resulting in inspired creativity for current projects and confident goal setting for the future.

Learn the movements of Xcelwellness Tai Chi and practice those moves until they feel quite comfortable. If you fully understand the theory and grasp the small but powerful aspects of each move, you will create significant personal benefits from your practice.


## Safety

- Every person has a different body, with different strengths, weaknesses, and injuries: listen to your body and go to your limit.

- During the movements, deep breaths are taken - if you feel dizzy at any point, return your breathing to normal.

- If you have a history of back pain, shoulder pain, or hip pain, be gentle and go to your limit. If you have knee pain, be careful to avoid any knee twisting. Always keep your knees pointing over your feet in any posture.

Disclaimer: The information contained in this book is intended for educational purposes only and is not a substitute for diagnosis or treatment by a licensed physician.

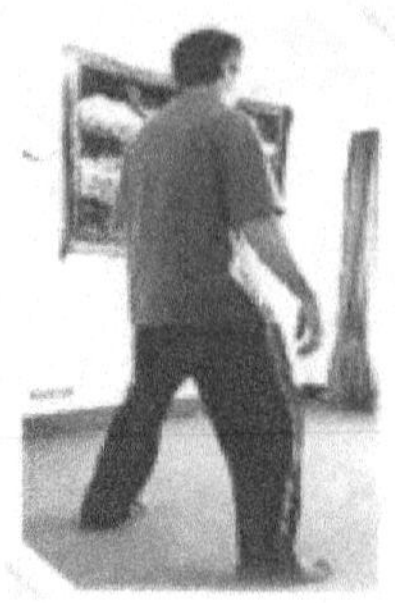

## Standing

In Tai Chi there is a special way to stand, as outlined below. This is called the parallel stance.

- Stand with feet shoulder-width apart, toes in line, and knees slightly bent in line with the direction of your feet.

- Imagine your head is elevated and you feel *suspended* from the crown. From there, relax your feet, relax your ankles, relax your knees, and feel as if your whole body is falling away from your head. Let your pelvis simply hang.

- Relax your spine. As they say in the ancient writings "let your spine hang like a string of pearls in the wind". From there your shoulders simply hang. Now, take a deep breath into your belly and see how relaxing this is.

## Breathing

Most of us breathe poorly. We take shallow breaths that keep us alive but do not allow us to thrive. The style of deep diaphragm breathing we will teach you and incorporate into the movements will help with better breathing techniques. As we breathe in through the nose, the belly expands; as we breathe out, the belly contracts forcing the air out. Breathe out through the nose or mouth.

How are you feeling after taking a few deep breaths? Energized, relaxed, focused, tingly, etc.

## Benefits of Deep Diaphragm Breathing:

- <u>Increases Relaxation</u>: Deep breathing produces a reflex called a 'Relaxation Response.' Taking a deep breath produces an almost instant state of relaxation.

- <u>Feeds our Cells</u>: Each of our cells performs a multitude of functions per second. Deep breathing provides the fuel they need to thrive while increasing our sense of vibrancy.

- <u>Improves Immune Function</u>: Lymph in our torso is a vital part of our immune system and it must move to be effective. It only moves if we move. Taking a deep breath, especially in conjunction with torso twisting, massages internal organs, moves lymph, and strengthens immunity.

## Core

Have you suffered from back pain? Most of us have a core that is lifeless and inflexible. But that can change with a Tai Chi secret that will help create a suppler core and a flexible spine.

Most of us move our spines in only two dimensions – up and down, forwards and backward. To dramatically improve spinal health, Xcelwellness Tai Chi will safely and gently rotate each vertebra. If you fix the bottom (don't let your bottom turn), fix the top (keep looking ahead), and rotate your shoulders under the chin, you will rotate every vertebra in your spine.

One of the best ways to age more gracefully is to become more flexible, both mentally and physically. Xcelwellness Tai Chi will increase the flexibility of your joints, especially your core and your spine.

## Patience

Sometimes people feel frustrated when they try to remember a series of movements. Sometimes your little internal voice says things like "You can't remember this", "you are too clumsy" or similar. It is vitally important to reframe this type of thinking. The key is to smile and to be persistent.

## Feeling Great

Each of our body's cells incorporates chemicals to perform a multitude of functions and keep us alive and active. Emotional states are influenced by neurochemicals. Feelings of love, happiness, and bliss are caused by internal chemical processes. The difference between positive and negative states of being is the amount of particular chemicals in circulation.

Xcelwellness Tai Chi movements help to decrease the negative chemicals surrounding your cells and increase the ones that will help you feel great. Understanding Tai Chi techniques will help you take charge of your feelings and of your life.

## Try this simple Exercise

Please close your eyes. Rate how you are feeling on a scale of one to ten, with one being "I am feeling poorly" and ten being "I feel so good!" Remember that number.

Now keeping your eyes closed, look up and smile for one whole minute.

Open your eyes and re-rate how you feel. Your number should be considerably higher.

## Stances in this Tai chi Course

The Balanced Stance: With the right foot at 45 degrees inwards, exhale and sink onto the right leg. With the left foot take a small step forward into a balanced stance, heel down first then flat foot.

The Cat Stance: The left foot is placed slightly behind the right foot in a cat stance (toes and the ball touching the floor.) This is the empty foot - 90% of the weight is on the right leg.

The Heel Stance: Exhale as the left foot lifts into a heel stance (heel touching floor only) and becomes an 'empty' foot. The weight is 70% on the rear leg.

The Parallel Stance: see next point.

## Standing Reminder for the Tai Chi Form

The parallel Stance: Standing in a parallel stance, facing north, feet shoulder-width apart, knees slightly bent over toes, and 'crown suspended from above.' Everything below relaxes, slightly sinking hip between legs.

Your head is elevated, and you feel *suspended* from the crown. From there, relax your feet, relax your ankles, relax your knees, and feel as if your whole body is falling away from your head. Remember to practice deep diaphragm breathing, smile, keep your chin up, and have fun in the Tai Chi Form.

# Warm-Up

## 1: The Rainbow Circle

This exercise stretches all parts of the body and massages the internal organs. Standing in a parallel stance, facing north, feet shoulder-width apart, knees slightly bent over toes, and 'crown suspended from above.' Everything below relaxes, slightly sinking hip between legs. If any muscle seems tight, focus on relaxing it; if necessary, shake it out.

Lift both arms, palms facing forward and parallel. Paint an imaginary 'rainbow circle' with your hands from left to right and down, bending your spine. Keep your legs straight, drop from the hip, and continue sweeping your hands back up around anticlockwise, slow, and easily, moving your whole body with suppleness to complete the full circle. Palms turn inward when bending forward on the downward curve of the circle. Inhale when painting the top of the circle and exhale when painting the bottom of the circle.

When you have 'painted' three times in this direction, pause and rest for a minute on the downward curve, relaxing your head, neck, shoulders, and arms. Hang loose like a goose.

Now, 'paint the rainbow circle' from right to left in the clockwise direction three times, slowly and easily, and finish at the original starting position with your hands at your sides.

## 2: Sawing Wood

This exercise encourages grounding and loosens up the torso, shoulders, and limbs. Standing in a parallel stance, facing north, feet shoulder-width apart, knees slightly bent over toes, and 'crown suspended from above.' Everything below relaxes, slightly sinking hip between legs. If any muscle seems tight, focus on relaxing it; if necessary, shake it out.

Take a step back with the right foot into a balanced stance. Then move your weight forward to the left leg and back to the right leg repeatedly as if you were cutting across a tree trunk with a two-person hand saw. Simultaneously, swing your arms from the shoulders back and forward with the rhythm generated. When your arms are back, squeeze your shoulder blades together to loosen the muscle fibers. Keep your hip relaxed, your feet flat and both knees slightly bent. Sit into the stance, so that your head and trunk do not bob up and down. Inhale on the backward swing and exhale on the forward swing. Repeat this momentum five times. Remember, slow and easy.

Then take a step back with the left foot into a balanced stance. Repeat this momentum five times on this side. Remember, slow and easy.

## 3: Moving the Ball

Standing in a parallel stance, facing north, feet shoulder-width apart, knees slightly bent over toes, and 'crown suspended from above.' Everything below relaxes, slightly sinking hip between legs. If any muscle seems tight, focus on relaxing it; if necessary, shake it out.

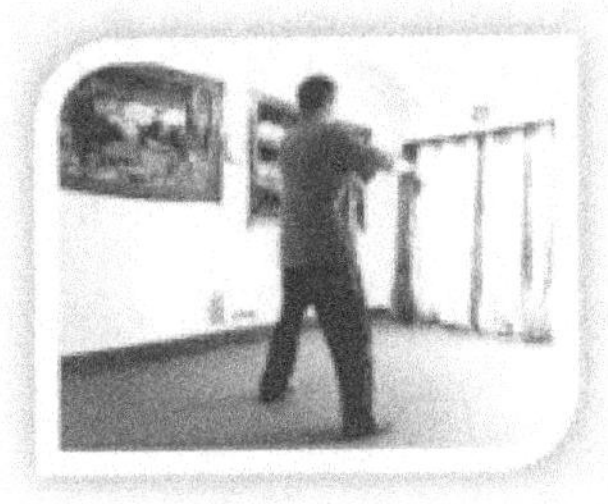

As one inhales, both hands (palms down) float up from the hip away from and in front of the body to shoulder height and then are slowly drawn toward the body and float back down during the exhale.

This exercise is performed three times in succession. The imagery in this warm-up is that from one's center (abdomen region), the hands float up effortlessly as if lifted up by an inflating balloon and then lower as if that balloon is deflating.

Deep diaphragm breathing is practiced so that during the inhale, air is drawn in to push the diaphragm down expanding the belly and filling the chest; and during the exhale, the belly contracts forcing the air out naturally without any strain. It is good to have a few seconds pause and hold between inhale and exhale movements to increase lung capacity and strength. Traditionally, air is drawn in through the nose and exhaled through either nose or mouth.

Moving the Ball is performed at the beginning and end of each practice session because it helps to center the practitioner in the here and now; to be present in the moment, still and aware of the internal and external.

# Section One: Ease and Relax

# Posture Set One: Grasping Sparrows Tail

<u>Rollback, Press, Push, and Single Whip</u>

Standing in a parallel stance, facing north, feet shoulder-width apart, knees slightly bent over toes, 'crown suspended from above.' Everything below relaxes, slightly sinking hip between legs. If any muscle seems tight, focus on relaxing it; if necessary, shake it out.

*Rollback: A:* Begin inhalation and move weight to the right, swivel the left foot to point 45 degrees NE. Move the weight back and sink on the supporting left leg, exhale, and take a step with the right leg and place into a balanced stance facing east. Simultaneously the right-hand sweeps around and points east in a 'handshake,' palm facing north, at chest height; the left hand is across the abdomen, palm facing inwards. Weight ends up 70% on the right foot; Eyes looking east.

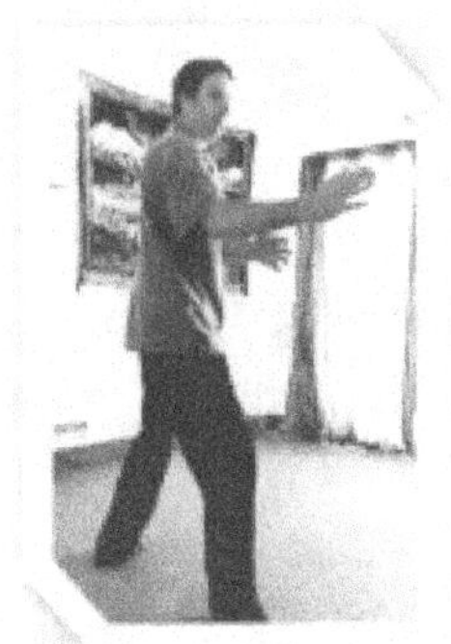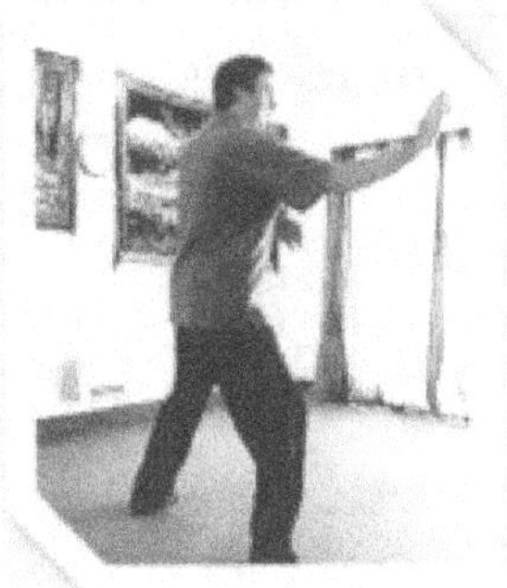

_B:_ Inhale and turn the torso to the right achieving a good safe stretch. The hands follow the move.

Turn back to the left diagonal (NE) and pause, pushing the right palm outward and away during an exhale as if to expel negative tension. Eyes following the movement. Weight ends up 70% on the right foot.

_C:_ Continue the torso turn to the left as far as one can safely go, inhaling, hands and eyes following, feet still, and careful with the knees. Left hand leading and away to the southwest, palm facing northward. The right arm across the chest ends up palm facing inwards. Exhaling, turn torso back to face the east, arms moving with the body.

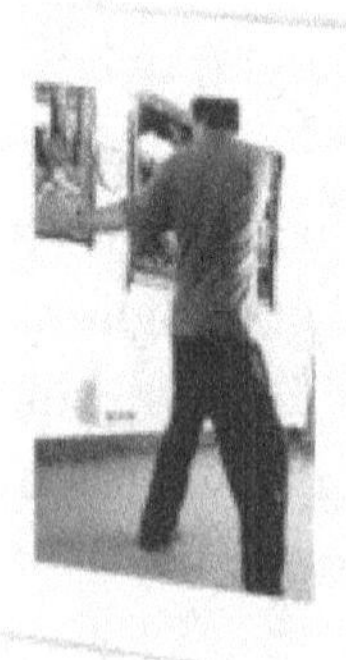

_Press: A: Left Palm Press:_ Inhale and lean weight back as palms join at waist height and sweep up to chest height, the left palm to press the right palm.

Exhale as the left palm pressed against the right palm pushes forward and away. The feet stay in position and weight ends up 70% on the front foot.

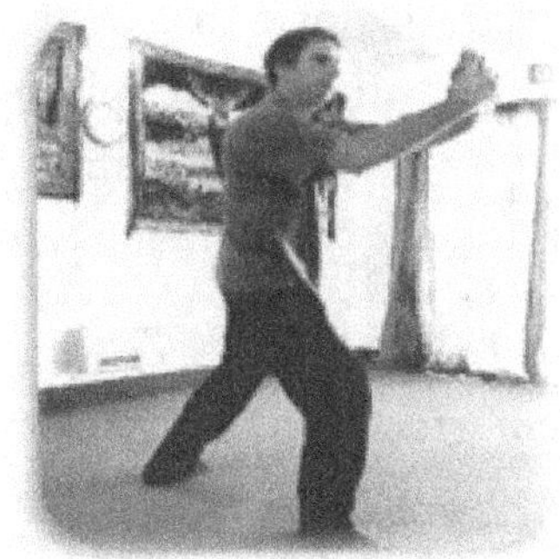

_B: Right Palm Press:_ Inhale and lean weight back as palms join at waist height and sweep up to chest height, right palm to press the left palm.

Exhale as the right palm pressed against the left palm pushes forward and away. The feet stay in position and weight ends up 70% on the front foot.

_Push:_ Inhale and lean the weight back as the hands separate (palms inward facing) and sweep in an arc up the center of the body from hip to shoulder height (imagine drawing positive energy up the body line).

Exhale as the torso and palms at shoulder height push forward and away (as if pushing an object). Your eyes follow the arc movement as weight settles 70% on the front foot.

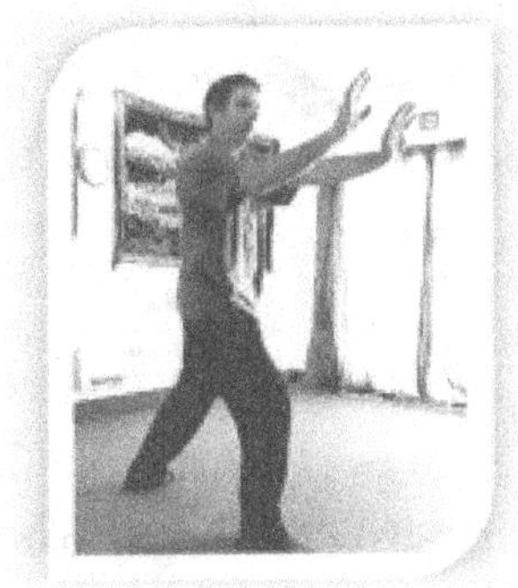

_Intermediary Roll-Back to left: A:_ Inhaling, turn the torso to the left as far as one can safely go, hands and eyes following. The feet are still and careful with the knees. Left hand leading the turn away to the southwest, palm ends facing northward. The right arm across the chest ends up palm facing inwards.

At full extension of the torso, arms, and shoulders, swivel the right foot 45 degrees inwards which facilitates an extra inch move of the extension into the left diagonal, effecting a good torso stretch.

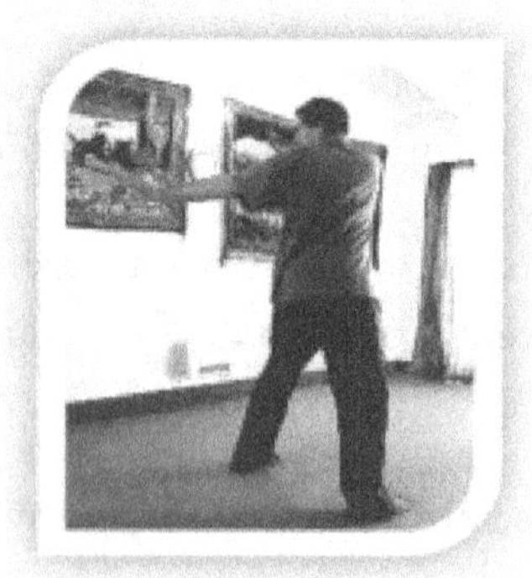 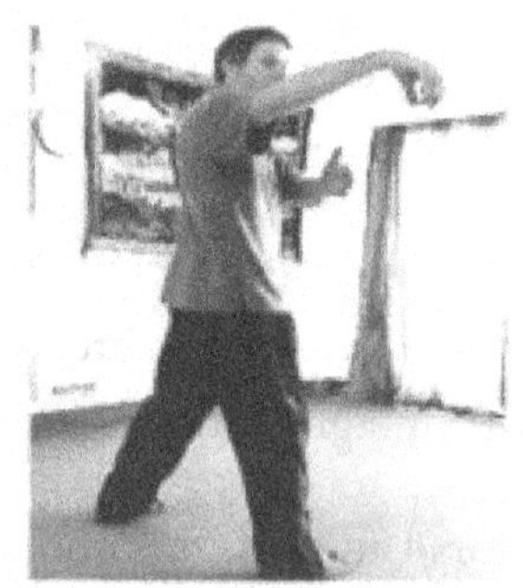

_B:_ Exhaling, turn the torso back to face the east, eyes and arms moving with the body turn. Halfway around, the right hand forms a hook hand (fingers and thumb touching with a bend in the wrist in the form of a hook). At full extension to the northeast, the left palm is at midriff height palm facing inward; the right 'hook hand' is extended toward the east. Feet stay in place in a balanced stance.

_Single Whip: A:_ Inhale and return to the west, eyes and left hand coming around, palm inward. The right hand is still extended in the 'hook hand' to the northeast corner.

Exhaling, sink onto the right leg (which is still at 45 degrees inwards), and with the left foot take a small step toward the west into a balanced stance, heel down first then flat foot. The left palm is at midriff height, a short distance from the body, palm facing inward. The right hand is still extended in the 'hook hand' to the northeast corner. Complete the movements in sync with the exhale.

_B:_ Facing west, inhale, and lean the body weight back as the left hand (palm inward facing) sweeps in an arc up the center of the body from the hip to shoulder height (imagine drawing positive energy up the body line).

Exhale as the torso and left palm at shoulder height push forward and away (as if pushing an object).

Your eyes follow your hand movement as the body weight settles 70% on the front foot. The right hand is still extended in the 'hook hand' to the northeast corner. Complete the movements in sync with the exhale.

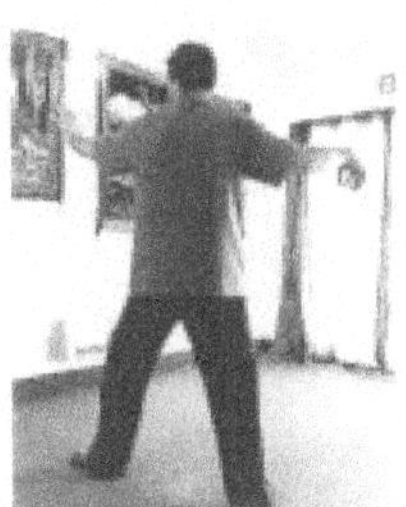

# Posture Set Two: Shoulder Stroke

## Lifting Hands, Shoulder Stroke

Standing in Single Whip, balanced stance, left foot forward, facing west, left palm at shoulder height forward and away. The right hand is at shoulder height in the 'hook hand' to the northeast corner.

*Lifting Hands: A:* Inhaling, raise the right heel off the floor in a cat stance (toes and the ball touching the floor. This is the empty foot - 90% of the weight is in the left leg). Simultaneously, release the right hook hand and bring both palms facing each other at shoulder height (imagine holding a ball). Eyes looking at the 'ball.'

*B:* Exhaling, sink into the left leg and lift and place the right foot slightly behind and to the right of the left foot in a cat stance (about 5cm gap and heel off the floor. This is the empty foot - 90% of the weight is in the left leg). Simultaneously, the torso and eyes turn to the southwest diagonal and both hands sweep down to hip height in front of the body, palms inwards.

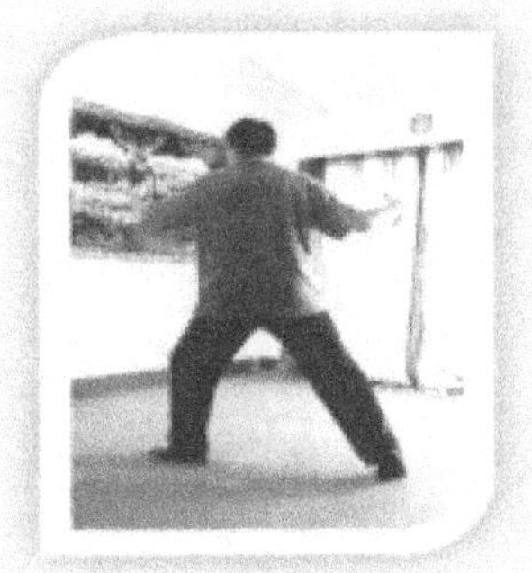 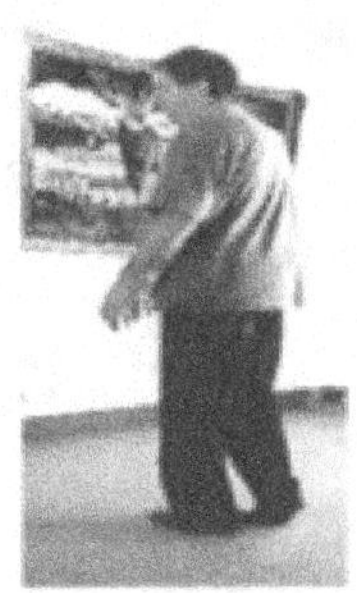

*Shoulder Stroke:* Inhaling, sink into the left leg, lift the right foot, and place it heel first, then flat, a good distance to the north into a balanced stance.

Exhale as 70% of the weight is moved to the right leg; the right hand settles in front of the hip, palm inwards, and the left palm is facing north at chest height. There is a good space between the legs and the eyes look north. This is a solid defensive warrior posture.

*Mini Shoulder Stroke:* Inhaling, sink into the right leg, lift the left foot, and place it slightly behind the right foot in a cat stance (toes and the ball touching the floor. This is the empty foot).

Exhale as 90% of the body weight remains on the right leg. The right hand remains in front of the hip, palm inwards, and the left palm remains facing north at chest height. The eyes look north.

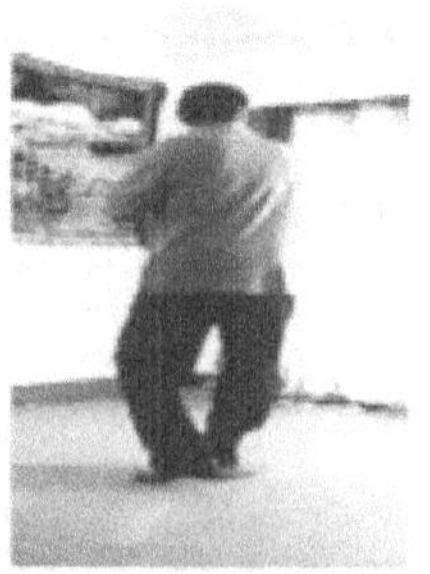
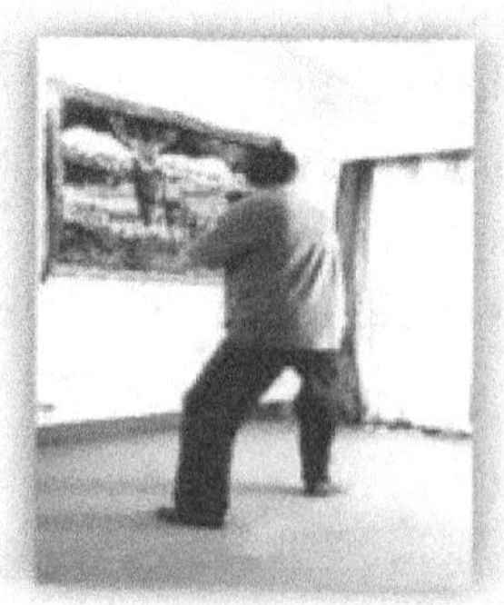

# Posture Set Three: Stork Cools Wings

<u>**Stork Cools Wings, Brush Left Knee**</u>

Standing in Mini-Shoulder Stroke: facing west, looking north. The left foot is placed slightly behind the right foot in a cat stance (toes and the ball touching the floor. This is the empty foot - 90% of the weight is on the right leg). The right hand is in front of the hip, palm inwards, and the left palm is facing north at chest height.

_Stork Cools Wings:_ Inhaling with the body weight on the right leg, lift the left foot and place it a good distance to the west into a cat stance (toes and the ball touching the floor. This is the empty foot - 90% of the weight is on the right leg).

Exhale as the body settles into this posture with the left palm downwards at the left hip; and the right palm facing outwards at forehead height (protecting the head). Keep the shoulders relaxed as the eyes look west with breathing in sync with movements.

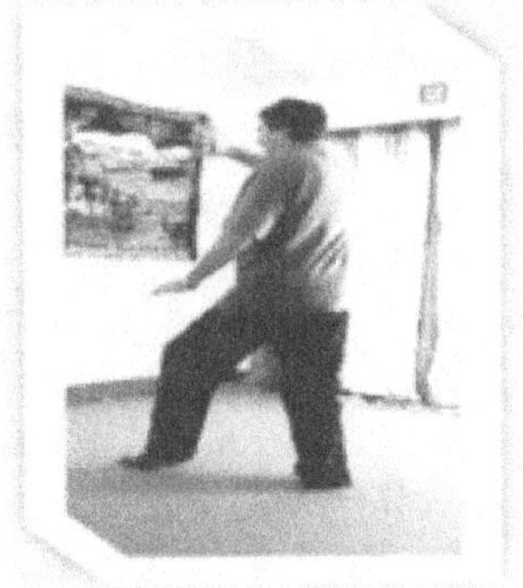

_Brush Left Knee:_ Inhaling, bring both palms toward each other at chest height (imagine holding a ball). Move this 'ball' back to the northeast diagonal effecting a good torso stretch with the eyes following the movement. As the weight moves backward, the left foot is flat on the floor.

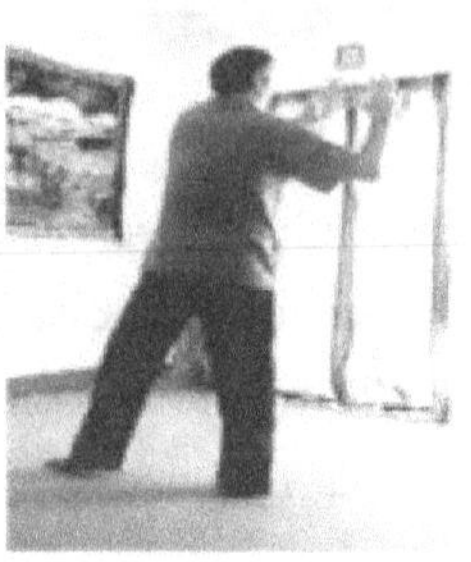 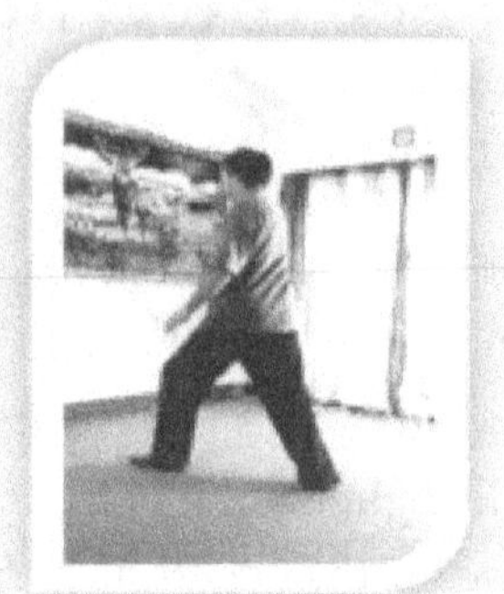

Exhaling, lift the left foot and place slightly forward as the weight moves back to the west and the 'ball' returns to center. The hands separate: the left palm brushes and settles downwards over the left thigh while the right palm pushes outwards and away at shoulder height. Both feet are flat in a balanced stance as movements are completed in sync with the breathing. The body weight is 70% on the left foot with eyes looking west.

# Posture Set Four: Punch Forward

## Punch Forward

Standing in Brush Left Knee, facing west, balanced stance, left foot forward, and the left palm facing downwards over the left thigh while the right palm faces outwards and away at shoulder height. Both feet are flat in a balanced stance. The weight is 70% on the left foot with eyes looking west.

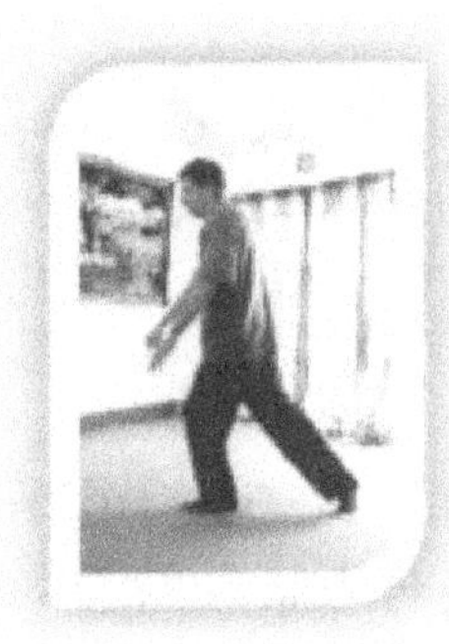

*Punch Forward: A:* Inhaling as the weight moves backward, draw the hands back to each frontal side of the thigh: left-hand palm facing inwards, while the right hand forms a light fist (which is held throughout the posture-set.) The torso, hands, and eyes turn left, and the left foot is empty to take a small step to the southwest corner, heel touches down first then the flat foot. Exhaling, the body weight moves forward onto the left leg, freeing up the right heel to peel off the floor for a few seconds as one sinks into this posture (appreciate this warrior stance). The hands are at each frontal side of the thigh: left-hand palm facing inwards; right hand in a fist.

*B:* Inhale as the right foot lifts off and the upper leg rises parallel with the floor, in the southwest corner briefly, before the whole frame skilfully swivels right to face the northwest corner. The right heel touches down first, then the flat foot.

Exhaling, the body weight moves forward onto the right leg, freeing up the left heel to peel off the floor for a few seconds as one sinks into this posture (appreciate this warrior stance). The hands are at each frontal side of the thigh: left-hand palm facing inwards; right hand in a fist.

*C:* Inhale as the torso, hands, and eyes turn left and the left foot is empty to take a good step to the west, heel touches down first, then the flat foot.

Exhaling the weight moves westward, 70% onto the left leg as the left palm faces inwards at belly height, and the right fist punches forward to the west at chest height.

# Posture Set Five: Push and Cross Hands

**<u>Push and Cross Hands</u>**

Standing in Punch Forward, facing west, balanced stance. The body weight is 70% on the left leg. The left palm faces inwards at belly height, and the right fist is extended in a punch forward to the west at chest height.

*<u>Push:</u>* Inhale, and lean the body weight back to the rear leg as both hands (palms inward facing) sweep in an arc up the center of the body from the hip to shoulder height (imagine drawing positive energy up the body line).

Exhale as the torso and palms at shoulder height push forward and away (as if pushing an object).

Your eyes follow the arc movement as the body weight settles 70% on the front foot.

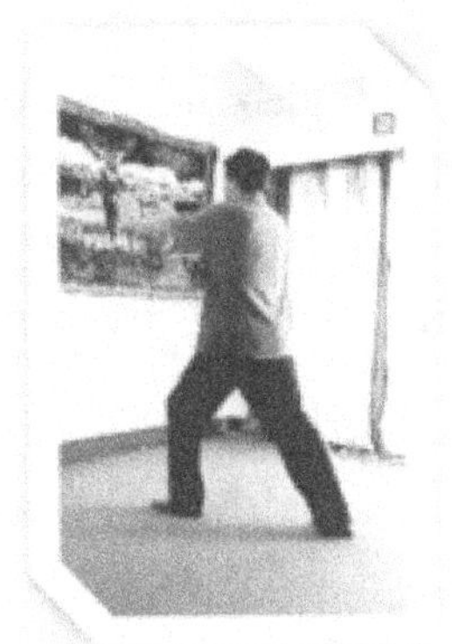 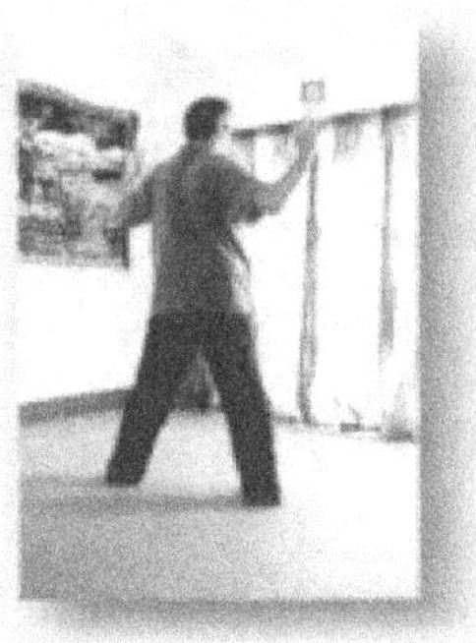

*Cross Hands: A:* Inhale as the torso turns to the right to face north with both hands turning to face north, palms outward facing at shoulder height. Simultaneously, the left foot swivels on the heel to face north while the right foot stays in place. The elbows can be moved backward to effect a shoulder blade squeeze for added measure.

*B:* Exhale as the right foot is freed up to turn and point north in a parallel stance, body weight evenly spread. Simultaneously, both wrists cross in front of the chest, palms inward facing and a short distance from the body.

(Imagine holding a ball of energy – contain the energy that you have cultivated during the posture sets.

Feel the internal. Be aware of the external. Relax the whole frame, suspended from above, and rooted to the earth through the feet.

This concludes Section One. If concluding your practice here, finish with Moving the Ball. Moving the Ball is a cool-down exercise.


## Moving The Ball

Standing in a parallel stance, facing north, feet shoulder-width apart, knees slightly bent over toes, 'crown suspended from above.' Everything below relaxes, slightly sinking hip between legs. If any muscle seems tight, focus on relaxing it; if necessary, shake it out.

As one inhales, both hands (palms down) float up from the hip away from and in front of the body to shoulder height and then are slowly drawn toward the body and float back down during the exhale.

This exercise is performed three times in succession. The imagery in this exercise is that from one's center (abdomen region) the hands float up effortlessly as if lifted up by an inflating balloon and then lower as if that balloon is deflating.

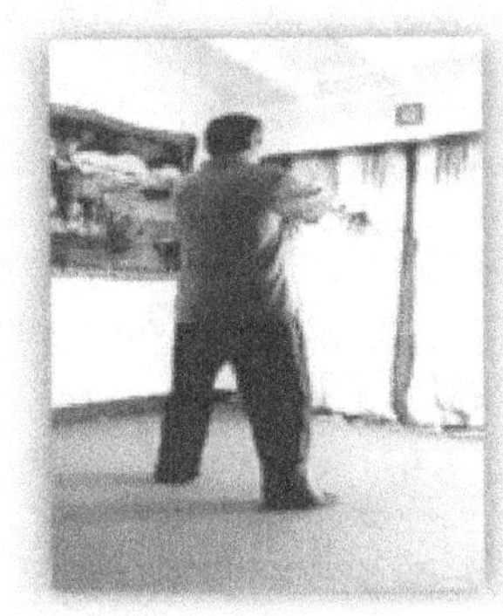

Deep diaphragm breathing is practiced so that during the inhale, air is drawn in to push the diaphragm down expanding the belly and filling the chest; and during the exhale, the belly contracts forcing the air out naturally without any strain. It is good to have a few seconds pause and hold between inhale and exhale movements to increase lung capacity. Traditionally, the air is drawn in through the nose and exhaled through either the nose or mouth.

This exercise is performed to begin and end each practice session because it helps to center the practitioner in the here and now; to be present in the moment, still, and aware of the internal and the external.

# Section Two: Cleanse and Instil

## Posture Set One: Grasping Sparrows Tail

### Rollback, Press, Push & Single Whip

Standing in a parallel stance, facing north, feet shoulder-width apart, knees slightly bent over toes, 'crown suspended from above.' Everything below relaxes, slightly sinking hip between legs. If any muscle seems tight, focus on relaxing it; if necessary, shake it out.

*Rollback: A:* Begin inhalation and move weight to the right, swivel the left foot to point 45 degrees NE. Move the weight back and sink on the supporting left leg, exhale, and take a step with the right leg and place into a balanced stance facing east. Simultaneously the right-hand sweeps around and points east in a 'handshake,' palm facing north, at chest height; the left hand is across the abdomen, palm facing inwards. Weight ends up 70% on the right foot; Eyes looking east.

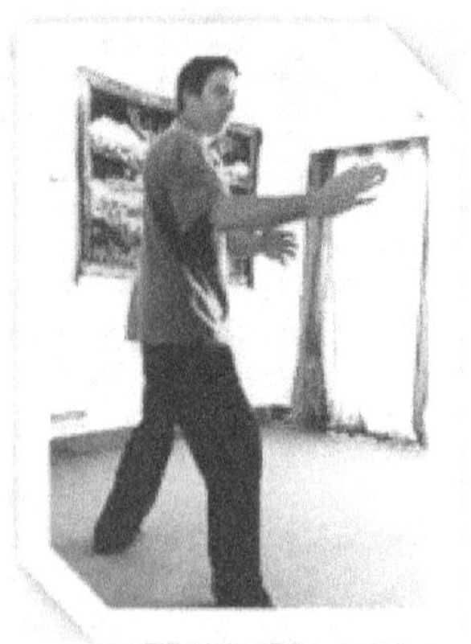
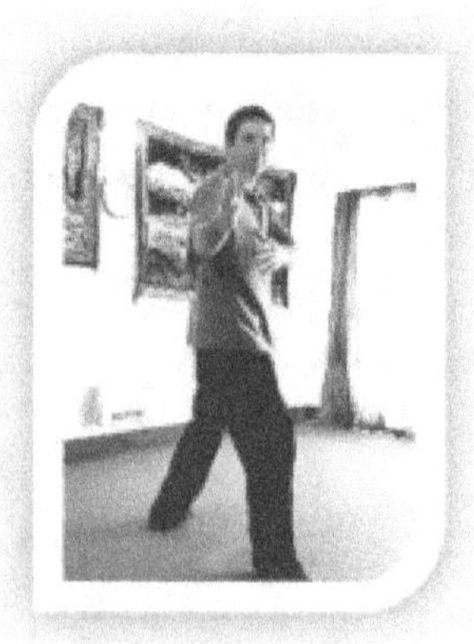

*B:* Inhale and turn the torso to the right achieving a good safe stretch. The hands follow the move.

Turn back to the left diagonal (NE) and pause, pushing the right palm outward and away during an exhale as if to expel negative tension. Eyes following the movement. Weight ends up 70% on the right foot.

*C:* Continue the torso turn to the left as far as one can safely go, inhaling, hands and eyes following, feet still, and careful with the knees. Left hand leading and away to the southwest, palm facing northward. The right arm across the chest ends up palm facing inwards.

Exhaling, turn torso back to face the east, arms moving with the body.

*Press: A: Left Palm Press:* Inhale and lean weight back as palms join at waist height and sweep up to chest height, the left palm to press the right palm.

Exhale as the left palm pressed against the right palm pushes forward and away. The feet stay in position and weight ends up 70% on the front foot.

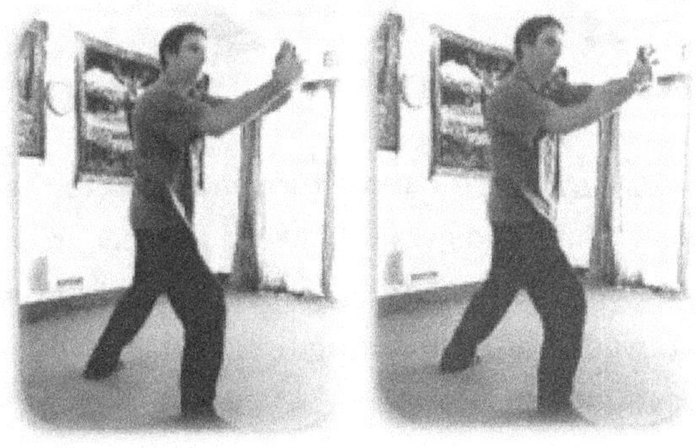

*B: Right Palm Press:* Inhale and lean weight back as palms join at waist height and sweep up to chest height, right palm to press the left palm.

Exhale as the right palm pressed against the left palm pushes forward and away. The feet stay in position and weight ends up 70% on the front foot.

*Push:* Inhale and lean the weight back as the hands separate (palms inward facing) and sweep in an arc up the center of the body from hip to shoulder height (imagine drawing positive energy up the body line).

Exhale as the torso and palms at shoulder height push forward and away (as if pushing an object). Your eyes follow the arc movement as weight settles 70% on the front foot.

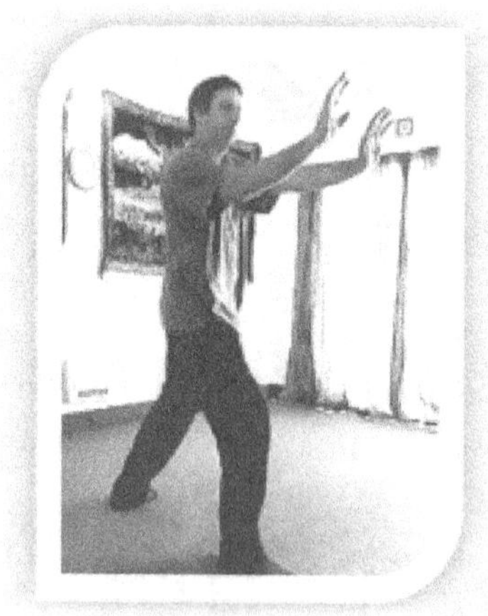 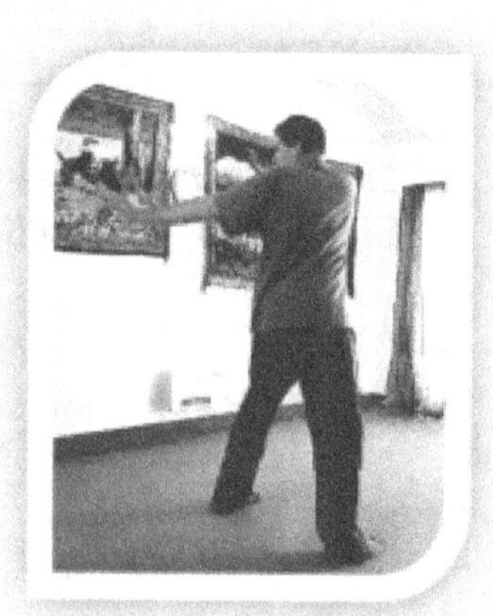

*Intermediary Roll-Back to left: A:* Inhaling, turn the torso to the left as far as one can safely go, hands and eyes following. The feet are still and careful with the knees. Left hand leading the turn away to the southwest, palm ends facing northward. The right arm across the chest ends up palm facing inwards.

At full extension of the torso, arms, and shoulders, swivel the right foot 45 degrees inwards which facilitates an extra inch move of the extension into the left diagonal, effecting a good torso stretch.

*B:* Exhaling, turn the torso back to face the east, eyes and arms moving with the body turn. Halfway around, the right hand forms a hook hand (fingers and thumb touching with a bend in the wrist in the form of a hook). At full extension to the northeast, the left palm is at midriff height palm facing inward; the right 'hook hand' is extended toward the east. Feet stay in place in a balanced stance.

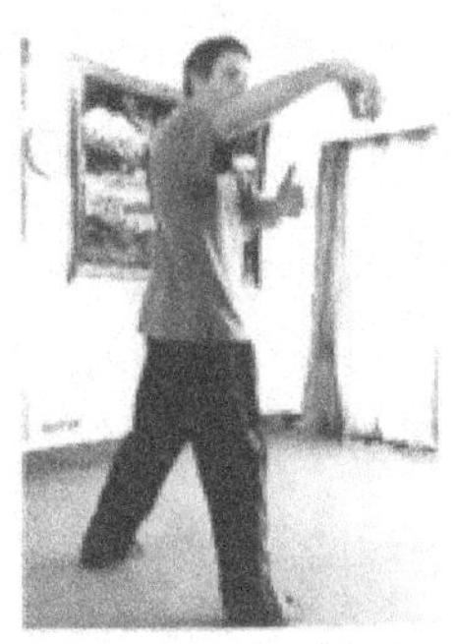 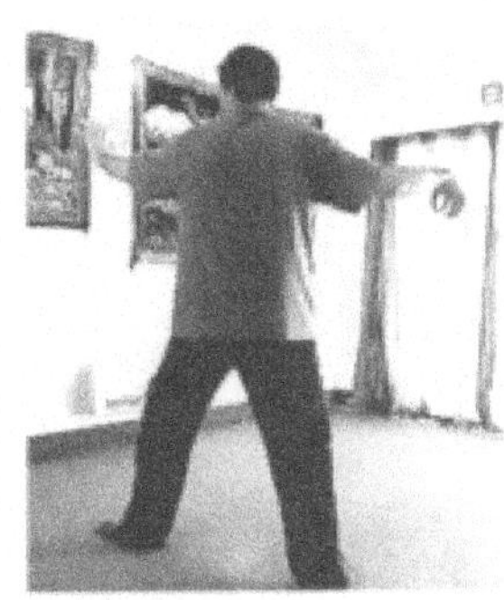

*Single Whip: A:* Inhale and return to the west, eyes and left hand coming around, palm inward. The right hand is still extended in the 'hook hand' to the northeast corner.

Exhaling, sink onto the right leg (which is still at 45 degrees inwards), and with the left foot take a small step toward the west into a balanced stance, heel down first then flat foot. The left palm is at midriff height, a short distance from the body, palm facing inward. The right hand is still extended in the 'hook hand' to the northeast corner. Complete the movements in sync with the exhale.

*B:* Facing west, inhale, and lean the body weight back as the left hand (palm inward facing) sweeps in an arc up the center of the body from the hip to shoulder height (imagine drawing positive energy up the body line).

Exhale as the torso and left palm at shoulder height push forward and away (as if pushing an object).

Your eyes follow your hand movement as the body weight settles 70% on the front foot. The right hand is still extended in the 'hook hand' to the northeast corner. Complete the movements in sync with the exhale.

# Posture Set Two: Repulse Monkey

## Punch Under Elbow, Repulse Monkey, Holding the Ball to the Left

Standing in Single Whip, in a balanced stance, left foot forward, facing west, left palm at shoulder height, forward and away, and right hand at shoulder height in a hooked hand to the northeast corner.

*Punch under Elbow: A:* Inhale as the weight moves onto the left leg. Lift and place the right leg forward, west, a good distance, heel first then a flat foot. Simultaneously, release the right hook hand and move the arm extended westward finishing open palm facing south. The left hand comes around with the torso, palm open facing south. Exhale as the body settles into this posture, eyes looking south, and the body weight evenly spread.

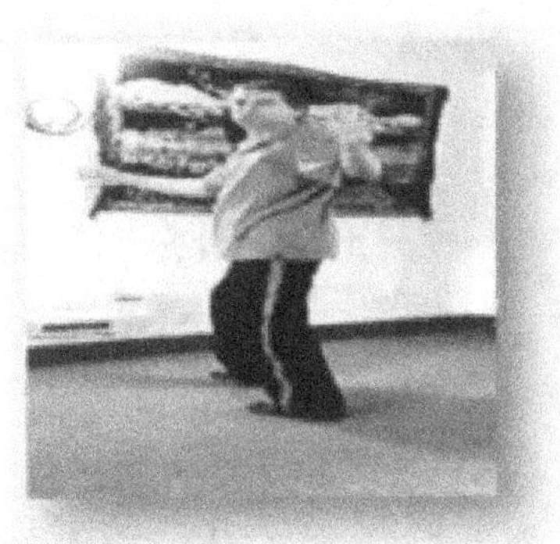
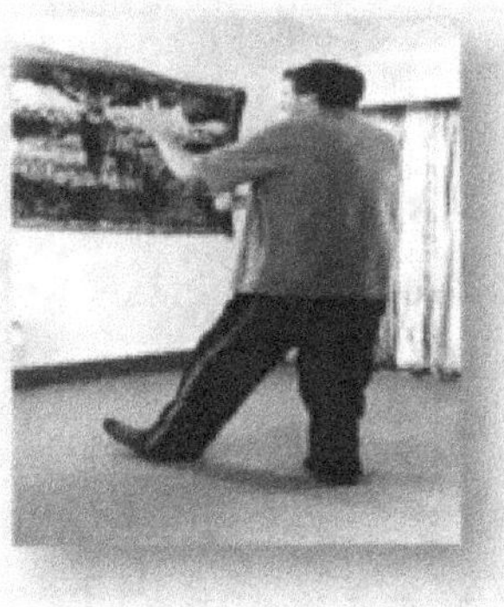

*B:* Inhale as the body weight moves back to the left leg, and the right leg lifts and places back into the original position, in a balanced stance, eyes and torso facing west. The left palm is at shoulder height facing north, elbow bent. The weight moves back onto the right foot.

Exhale as the left foot lifts into a heel stance (heel touching floor only) and becomes an 'empty' foot. The weight is 70% on the rear leg. The right hand forms a light fist positioned horizontally near the left elbow.

*Repulse Monkey: A:* Inhaling, the torso and eyes turn right to the north. The left foot is placed flat pointing into the Northwest corner. Simultaneously, both hands follow the movement winding up shoulder height, palms open facing north. The right foot stays in place, weight even.

*B:* Exhaling, the torso and eyes move back left to face the west, the left foot coming back to a balanced stance. The left hand rests palm up at hip height, while the right hand, at shoulder height, has the palm facing out and away toward the west. The body weight settles evenly, shoulders and hips relaxed as the exhale is complete.

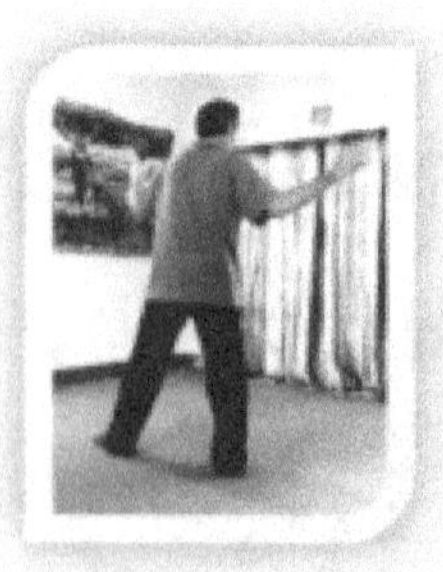 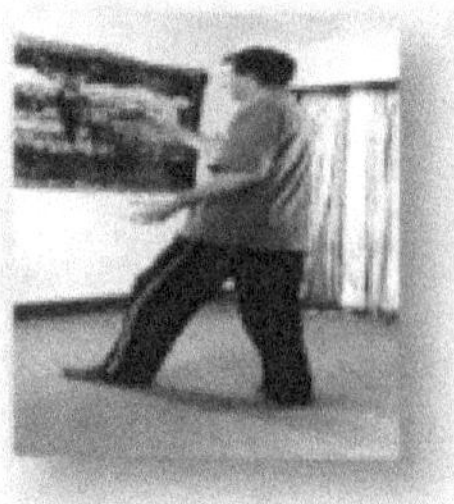 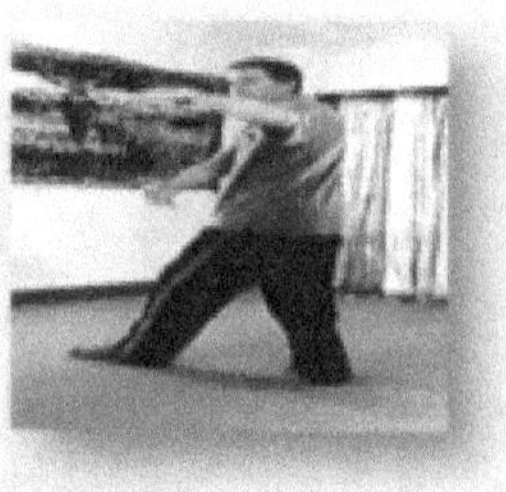

*Holding the Ball to the Left:* Inhale as the weight moves to the left leg, torso, and eyes turn left to face south, keeping both feet in place. The left hand is at shoulder height palm facing down; the right hand is at belly height palm facing up (imagine holding a ball). The action is like winding up a spring to unleash in the next move.

(The exhale and moves are shown in the next Posture-set).

# Posture Set Three: Diagonal Flying

## Diagonal Flying, Wave Hands in Clouds

Standing in Holding the Ball to the Left, in a balanced stance, the weight is on the left leg, torso, and eyes face south. The left hand is at shoulder height, palm facing down; the right hand is at belly height, palm facing up (imagine holding a ball). The action is like winding up a spring to unleash in the next move. An inhalation is taken.

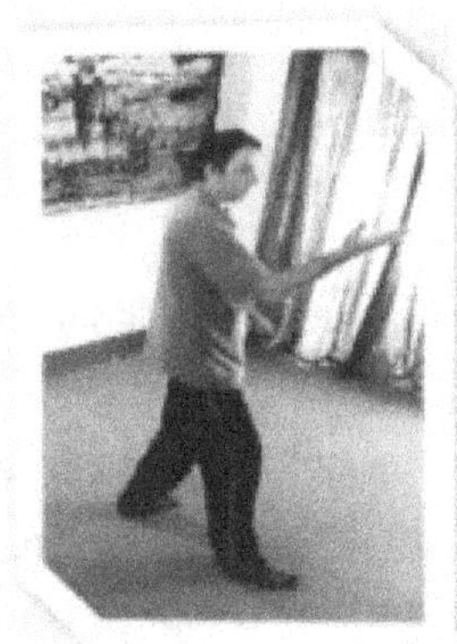

*Diagonal Flying:* Exhale as the torso sweeps to the right to face Northeast. The left foot swivels on the heel 45 degrees inwards. The weight transfers to the left foot freeing up the right foot to swivel 45 degrees outward pointing Northeast, in a balanced stance. This movement occurs smoothly, with no stepping. Simultaneously, the hands sweep around, the right hand at forehead height, palm up, fingers pointing to the stars in the northeast corner. The eyes look up and past the fingers. The left hand is at hip height, palm facing inward. Complete the exhale in sync with the movements.

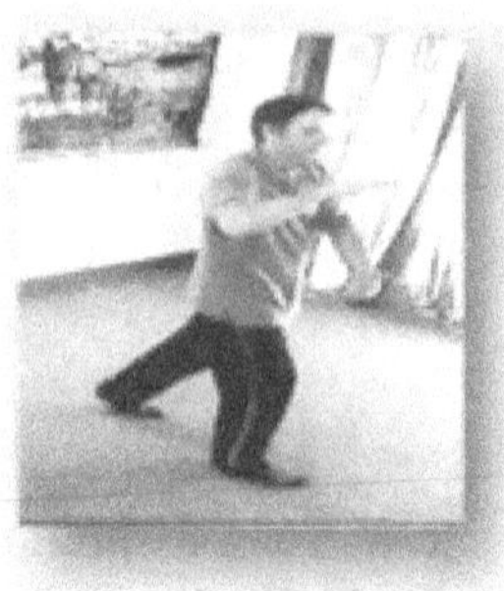

_Wave Hands in Clouds: A:_ Inhale as the weight shifts 70% to the right front leg. The left foot heel raises off the floor. Both hands are front and center, a distance from the body, holding the ball. The right palm is on top facing down; the left palm is on the bottom facing up. Exhale as you sink into the posture.

_B:_ Inhale as the left foot raises and places down shoulder width apart in line with the right foot in a parallel stance, weight even. Simultaneously, the hands exchange places past each other so that the right palm finishes on the bottom facing down at belly height, and the left palm is on top facing up at shoulder height. The legs are a good distance apart. Sink the pelvis between the legs, slight bend in the legs, relaxed and smooth movements in sync with breathing.

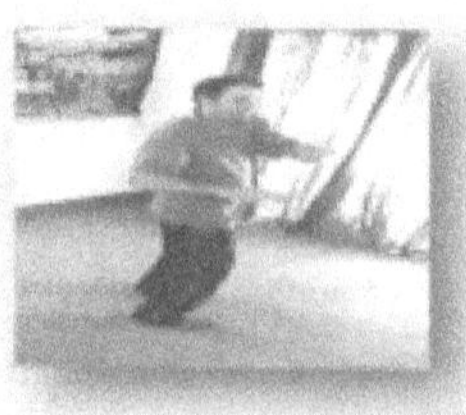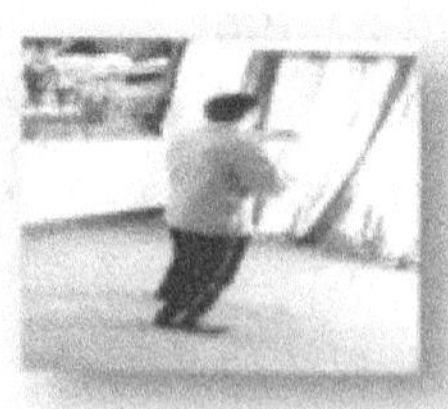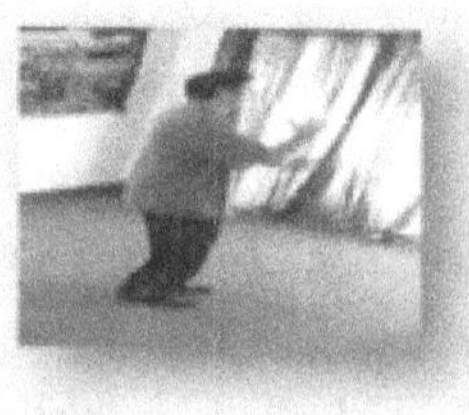

_C:_ Exhale as the weight and torso turn to the left. The hands stay in front of the body, wrists, and palms swivel so that by the time the full extension to the left is reached the hands are holding the ball again. The left palm is on top facing down at shoulder height; the right palm is on the bottom facing up at belly height. Complete the exhale in sync with the movements.

_D:_ Inhale as the right foot is empty to lift and slowly place a few inches beside the left foot. Remember to sink and place the foot. Simultaneously, the hands exchange places past each other so that the left palm finishes on the bottom facing down at belly height, and the right palm is on the top facing up at shoulder height. Maintain relaxed and smooth movements in sync with breathing.

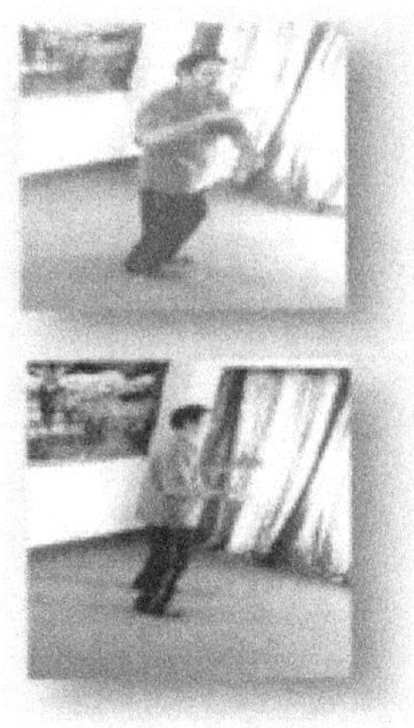

_E:_ Exhale as the weight and torso turn to the right. The hands stay in front of the body, wrists, and palms swivel so that by the time the full extension to the right is reached the hands are holding the ball again. The right palm is on top facing down at shoulder height; the left palm is on the bottom facing up at belly height. Complete the exhale in sync with the movements. This is ONE Wave Hands completed. Perform TWO more beginning with number _B_.

In Wave Hands in Clouds, one moves toward the northwest diagonal and eyes keep looking center.

_F:_ After the third Wave Hands is complete, during the exhale, the weight is moved back to the center facing the northeast corner. The hands finish in front of the body: left palm facing right at chest height and right palm facing left at belly height.

# Posture Set Four: Rooster On One Leg

**<u>Rooster on One Leg, Toe Kick (right side, then left side)</u>**

Standing in Wave Hands in Clouds, exhale completely. The weight is centered, facing the northeast corner. The hands are in front of the body: the left palm facing right at chest height, and the right palm is facing left at belly height.

*Rooster on One Leg, Right Side: A:* Inhale as the weight moves to the left leg, freeing up the right leg to lift up as high as is comfortable. Remember to sink into the supporting leg to aid balance, but keep the torso upright. The foot is relaxed down. Simultaneously, the right hand rises up to chest height in sync with the right leg (as if the hand is pulling the leg up), and the left palm settles at left hip height, facing inwards. Exhale as this position is held.

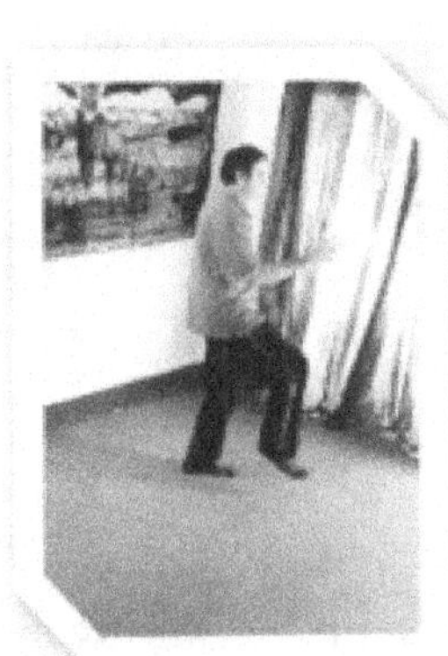
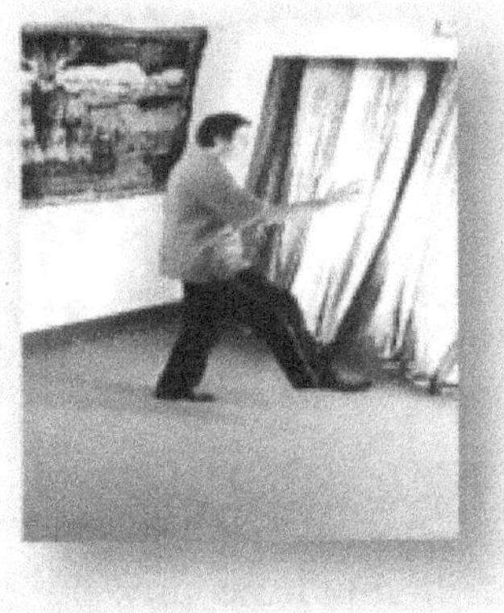

*Right Toe Kick: A:* Inhale as the right foot raises and gracefully kicks forward, toes pointed. Simultaneously, the hands separate in distance in this action. The right palm facing to the left follows the right leg movement, while the left hand backs off at hip height, palm facing inward. Remember to perform movements smoothly in sync with breathing and keep the torso upright.

*B:* Exhale as the right foot and hands return to the original position. Pause and then place the right foot directly back behind 45 degrees outward in a balanced stance.

*Rooster on One Leg, Left Side: A:* Inhale as the weight moves to the right leg, freeing up the left leg to lift up as high as is comfortable. Remember to sink into the supporting leg to aid balance, but keep the torso upright. The foot is relaxed down. Simultaneously, the left hand rises up to chest height in sync with the left leg (as if the hand is pulling the leg up); and the right palm settles at right hip height facing inwards. Exhale as this position is held.

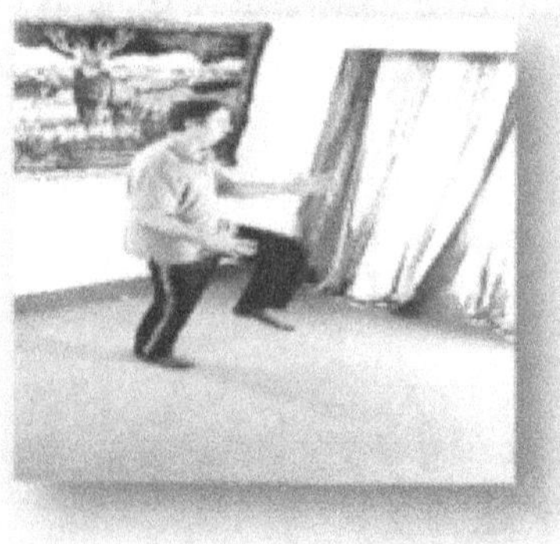
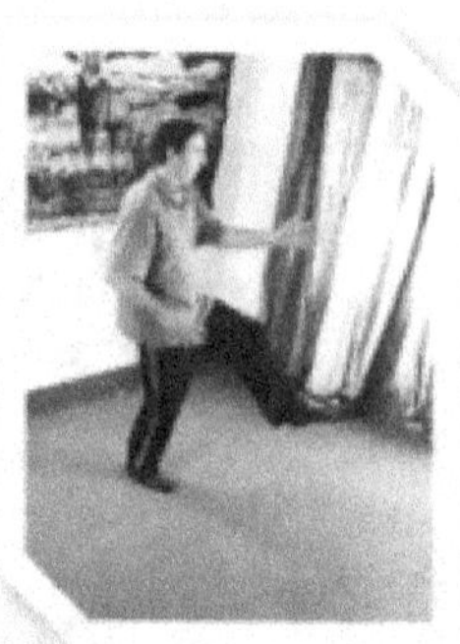

*Left Toe Kick: A:* Inhale as the left foot raises and gracefully kicks forward, toes pointed. Simultaneously, the hands separate in distance in this action, the left palm facing to the right follows the left leg movement, while the right hand backs off at hip height, palm facing inward. Remember to perform movements smoothly in sync with breathing and keep the torso upright.

_B:_ Begin the exhale as the left foot and hands return to the original position. Pause.

# Posture Set Five: Iron Fan

## Iron Fan, Turn Body & Chop

Standing in Rooster on One Leg, Left Side (after completing left Toe Kick), facing northeast. The weight is on the right leg freeing up the left leg to raise as high as is comfortable. Remember to sink into the supporting leg to aid balance, but keep the torso upright. The foot is relaxed down. The left palm is at chest height facing right, and the right palm settles at the right belly height, facing left. An inhalation is taken.

*Iron Fan:* Continue the exhale as the weight sinks into the right leg and the left foot is placed forward into a balanced stance. Simultaneously, the right hand rises up to ear height, palm facing outwards to the right; while the left palm is at chest height, extended in front, facing away and forward. Remember to perform movements smoothly in sync with the exhale finishing facing northeast and keep the torso upright.

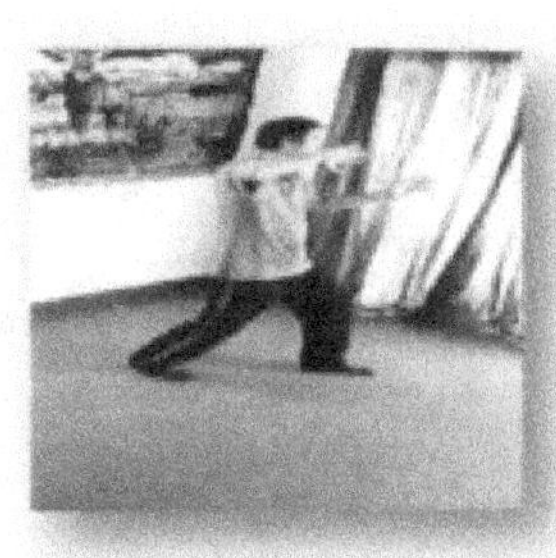

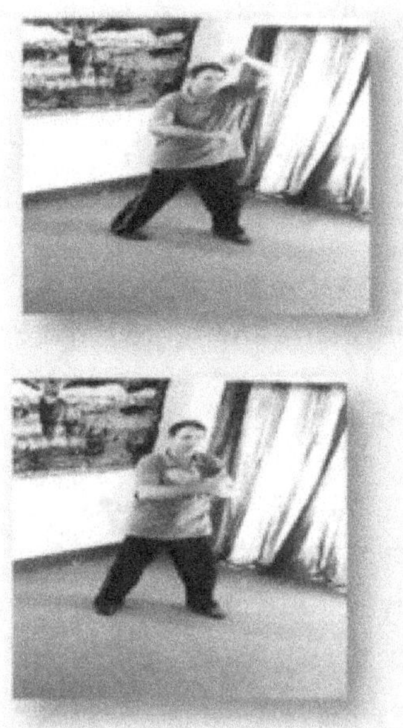

_Turn Body and Chop:_ Inhale as the whole body turns to the right facing east. The left foot swivels on the heel to point east, while the right foot stays in place. The right hand finishes a distance from the belly, palm facing downwards. The left palm facing outwards is at center forehead height. This is a defensive stance. Remember to keep the shoulders relaxed and sink the pelvis between the legs with a slight bend in the knees. The body weight is evenly spread. The exhale comes with the completion of Turn Body and Chop.

From here, if one continues into Section Three, then jump to Section 3A.

If one is concluding the practice session here, then complete the following movements of Cross Hands and Moving the Ball.

## Cross Hands

Facing East, exhale as the right foot is freed up to turn and point east in a parallel stance. The body weight is evenly spread. Simultaneously, both wrists cross in front of the chest, palms inward facing and a distance from the body.

(Imagine holding a ball of energy – contain the energy that you have cultivated during the Tai Chi Form thus far).

Feel the internal. Be aware of the external. Relax the whole frame, suspended from above and rooted to the earth through the feet.

## Moving The Ball

Standing in a parallel stance, facing east, feet shoulder-width apart, knees slightly bent over toes, 'crown suspended from above.' Everything below relaxes, slightly sinking hip between the legs. If any muscle seems tight, focus on relaxing it; if necessary, shake it out.

As one inhales, both hands (palms down) float up from the hip away from and in front of the body to shoulder height and then are slowly drawn toward the body and float back down during the exhale.

This exercise is performed three times in succession.

The imagery in this exercise is that from one's center (abdomen region), the hands float up effortlessly as if lifted up by an inflating balloon and then lower as if that balloon is deflating.

Deep diaphragm breathing is practiced so that during the inhale, air is drawn in to push the diaphragm down expanding the belly and filling the chest; and during the exhale, the belly contracts forcing the air out naturally without any strain. It is good to have a few seconds pause and hold between inhale and exhale movements to increase lung capacity. Traditionally, air is drawn in through the nose and exhaled through either the nose or mouth.

This exercise is performed to begin and end each practice session because it helps to center the practitioner in the here and now; to be present in the moment, still, and aware of the internal and external.

# Section Three: Energize and Empower

If continuing from Section Two, we complete Turn Body and Chop. Standing in a parallel stance, facing east, the left foot points east while the right foot points northeast. The right hand is at a distance from the belly, palm facing downwards. The left palm facing outwards is at center forehead height. This is a defensive stance. Remember to keep the shoulders relaxed and sink the pelvis between the legs with a slight bend in the knees. The body weight is even.

Exhale as the torso turns right to face the south. The weight moves onto the left leg freeing up the right leg to swivel on the heel to point south, in a balanced stance (a small step may be taken). The hands follow the movement: the right palm facing east comes to chest height, while the left palm facing west is at midriff height.

This then sets one up in the 'handshake' position to go into Grasping Sparrows Tail.

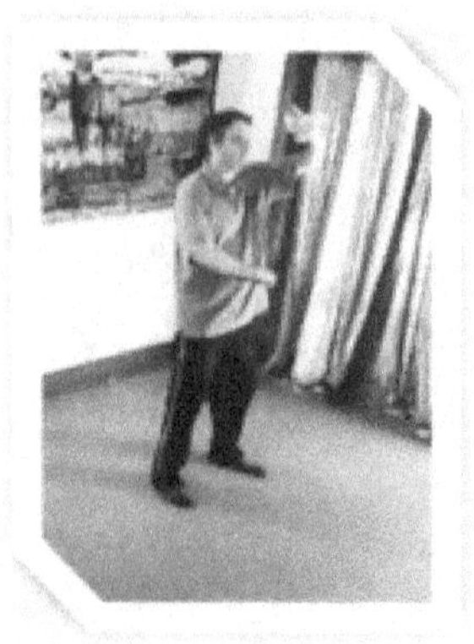 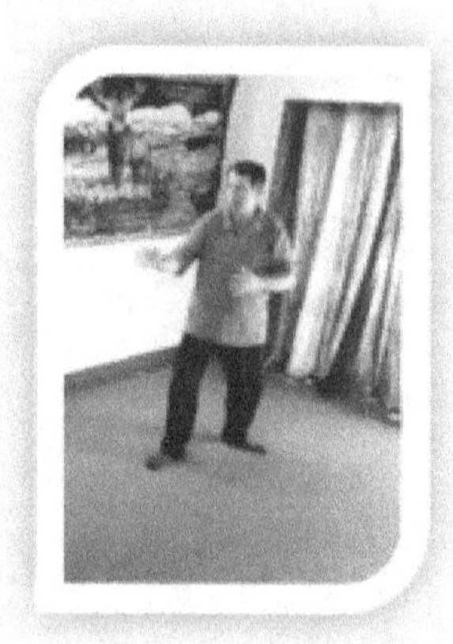

# Posture Set One: Grasping Sparrows Tail

## Rollback, Press, Push and Single Whip

Standing in a balanced stance, facing south, the right palm facing east comes to chest height, while the left palm facing west, is at midriff height. This then sets one up in the 'handshake' position to go into Grasping Sparrows Tail. Weight ends up 70% on the right foot. Eyes looking south.

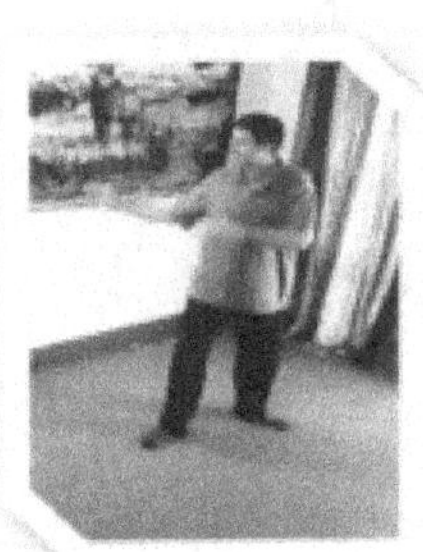
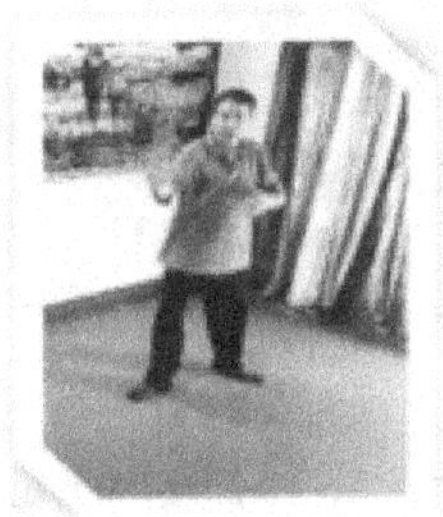
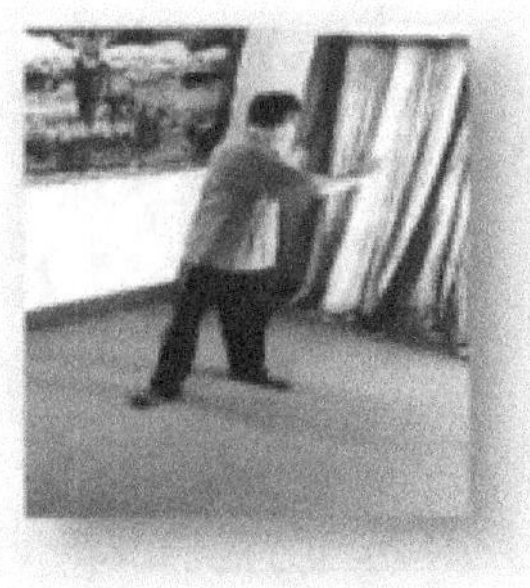

*Rollback: A:* Inhale and turn the torso to the right achieving a good safe stretch. Hands follow the move. Turn back to the left diagonal (SE) and pause, pushing the right palm outward and away during an exhale as if to expel negative tension. Eyes follow the movement. The body weight ends up 70% on the right foot.

*B:* Continue the torso turn to the left as far as one can safely go, inhaling, hands and eyes following, feet still, and careful with the knees. The left hand leads to the northeast. The left palm ends facing upward. The right arm across the chest ends up palm inwards and down facing.

Exhaling, turn the torso back to face the south, arms moving with the body.

*Press: A: Left Palm Press:* Inhale and lean the body weight back as palms join at waist height and sweep up to chest height, the left palm to press the right palm.

Exhale as the left palm pressed against the right palm pushes forward and away. The feet stay in position and the weight ends up 70% on the front foot.

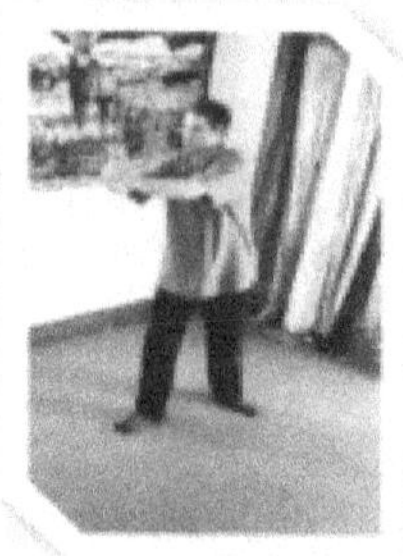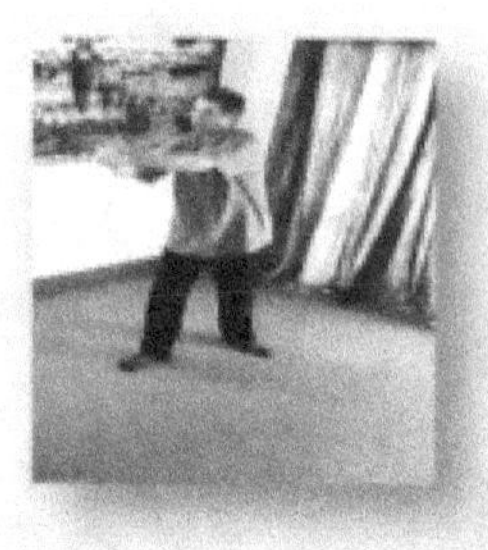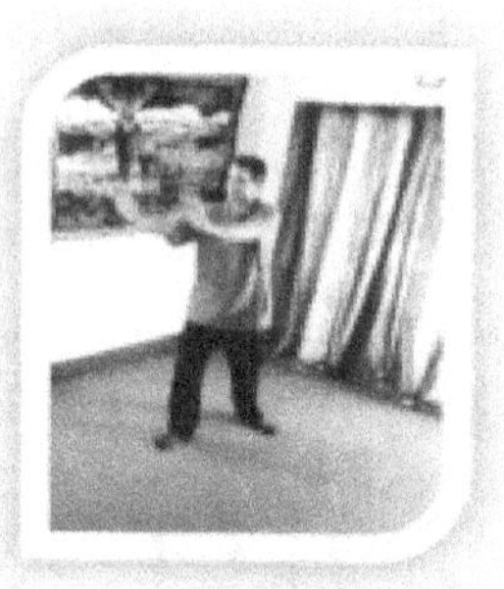

*B: Right Palm Press:* Inhale and lean the body weight back as palms join at waist height and sweep up to chest height, the right palm presses the left palm.

Exhale as the right palm pressed against the left palm pushes forward and away. The feet stay in position and the body weight ends up 70% on the front foot.

*Push:* Inhale and lean the body weight back as hands separate (palms inward facing) and sweep in an arc up the center of the body from hip to shoulder height (imagine drawing up positive energy).

Exhale as the torso and palms at shoulder height push forward and away (as if pushing an object).

Your eyes follow the arc movement as weight settles 70% on the front foot.

_Intermediary Roll-Back to left: A:_ Inhaling, turn the torso to the left as far as one can safely go, hands and eyes following, feet still, and careful with the knees. The left hand leads to the northeast, palm ends facing upward. The right arm across the chest ends up palm inwards and down facing.

At full extension of the torso, arms, and shoulders, swivel the right foot 45 degrees inwards which facilitates an extra inch move of the extension into the left diagonal, achieving a good torso stretch.

_B:_ Exhaling, turn the torso back to face the south, eyes, and arms moving with the body. Halfway around the right hand forms a hook hand (elbow bent, fingers and thumb touching, with a bend in the wrist to form a hook). At full extension to the southeast, the left palm is at midriff height, the palm facing inward. The right 'hook hand' is extended toward the south. The feet stay in place in a balanced stance.

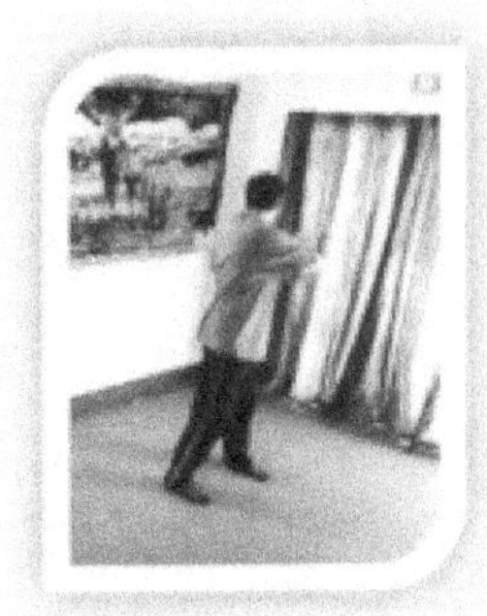 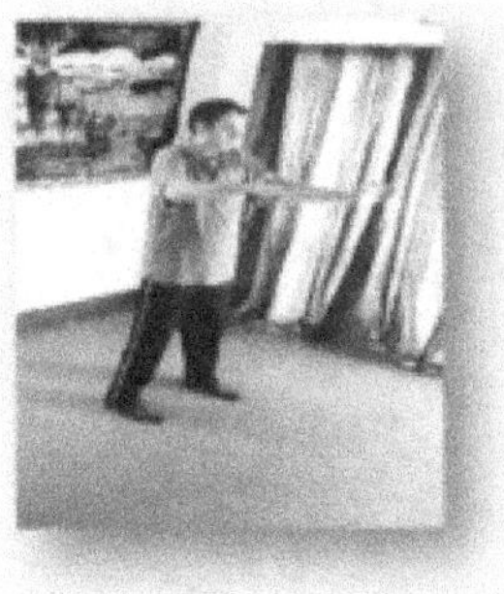 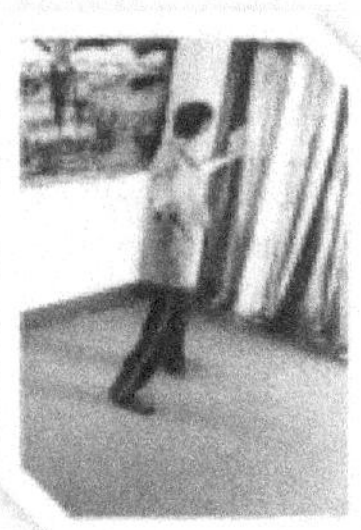

_Single Whip: A:_ Inhale and return to the north, eyes and the left hand coming around, palm inward. The right hand is still extended in the 'hook hand' to the southeast corner.

Exhaling, sink onto the right leg (which is still at 45 degrees inwards), and with the left foot, take a small step toward the north into a balanced stance, heel down first then flat foot. The left palm is at midriff height, a distance from the body, palm facing inward. The right hand is still extended in the 'hook hand' to the southeast corner. Complete the movements in sync with the exhale.

_B:_ Facing north, inhale, and lean the body weight back as the left hand (palm inward facing) sweeps in an arc up the center of the body from hip to shoulder height (imagine drawing up positive energy).

Exhale as the torso and left palm at shoulder height push forward and away (as if pushing an object).

Your eyes follow your hand movement as the body weight settles 70% on the front foot. The right hand is still extended in the 'hook hand' to the southeast corner. Complete the movements in sync with the exhale.

# Posture Set Two: Fair Lady Weaves the Shuttle

**<u>Fair Lady Weaves the Shuttle</u>**

Standing in Single Whip, balanced stance with 70% weight on the left foot forward, facing north. The left arm is extended, elbow bent, left palm at shoulder height pushed forward and away (as if pushing an object). The right hand is extended with the elbow bent in the 'hook hand' to the southeast corner.

*Fair Lady Weaves the Shuttle*:

*<u>To South East: A:</u>* Inhale as the torso turns right to face the south: the weight moves first onto the right leg to free up the left foot to swivel 45 degrees inwards, and then the weight moves onto the left leg, freeing up the right leg to swivel on the heel to point south, in a balanced stance (a small step may be taken). The hands follow the movement. The right palm facing east, comes to chest height, while the left palm facing west is at midriff height. This then sets one up in the 'handshake' position to go into Fair Lady Weaves the Shuttle.

Exhale as you settle into the posture.

*<u>B:</u>* Inhale as 70% of the body weight moves to the front foot. The fingers of the left hand point toward the open palm of the right hand. The left heel lifts off the floor and pauses.

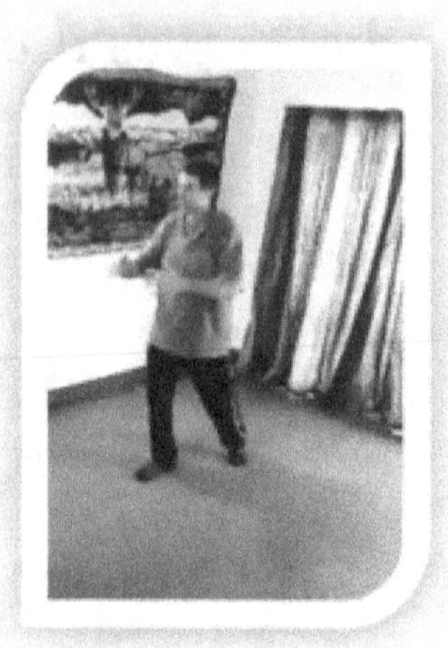 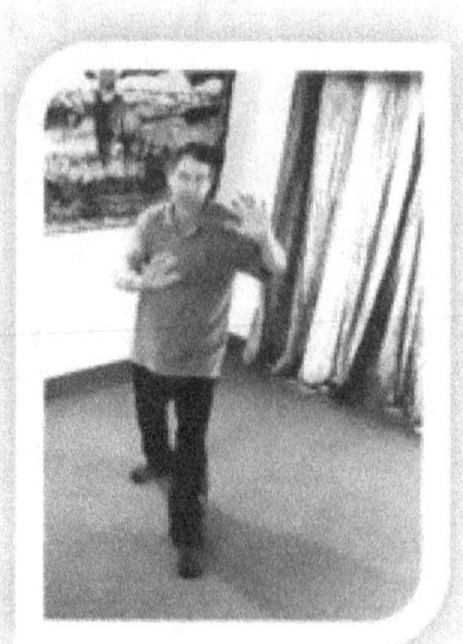

*C:* Exhale as the left foot steps forward toward the southeast corner into a balanced stance (remember to sink and place the foot). Weight moves 70% onto the left foot. Simultaneously, the left palm facing out and away finishes at face height with shoulders relaxed. The right palm is facing out and away at chest height. Complete the exhale in sync with movements.

*Transition to the west:* Inhale as the torso and hands turn right to the west direction swivelling on the heels to a balanced stance (a small step with the right foot may be taken). The weight is 70% on the front foot, and the left heel lifts off the floor and pauses. The palms are facing each other at chest height, and the fingers of the left hand are pointing at the open palm of the right hand.

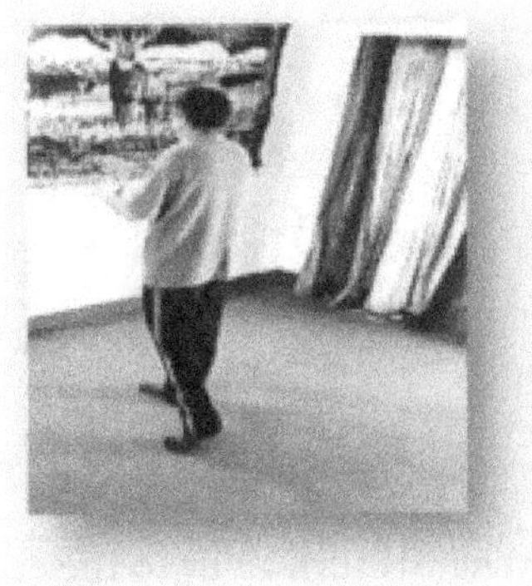 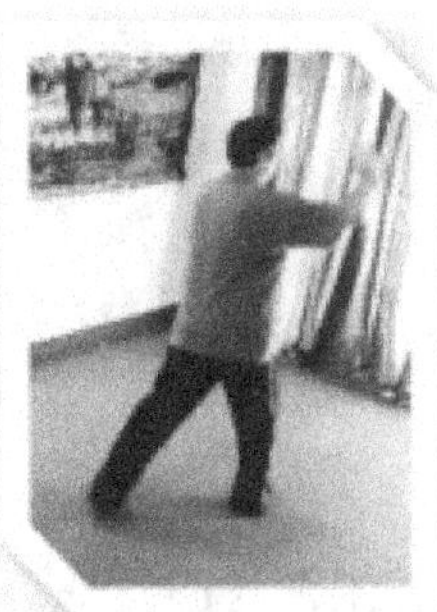

_To Northeast:_ Exhale as the weight moves back to the left leg. The torso turns right, the right leg lifts and steps to face the northeast corner, heel down first, then flat foot, while the left foot swivels 45 degrees to maintain a balanced stance. Seventy percent of the weight is on the right front foot. Simultaneously, the right palm facing out and away finishes at face height with shoulders relaxed. The left palm is facing out and forward at chest height.

Complete the exhale in sync with movements.

_To Northwest:_ A: Inhaling, the weight is 70% on the right front foot. The fingers of the left hand point toward the open palm of the right hand. The left heel lifts off the floor and pauses.

_B:_ Exhale as the left foot steps forward toward the northwest corner into a balanced stance (remember to sink and place the foot). The weight moves 70% onto the left foot. Simultaneously, the left palm facing out and away finishes at face height with shoulders relaxed. The right palm is facing out and away at chest height. Complete the exhale in sync with movements.

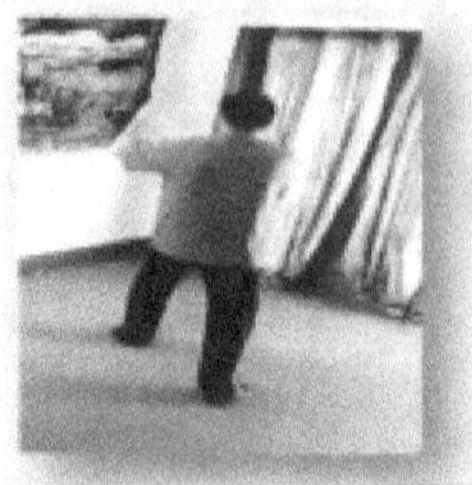 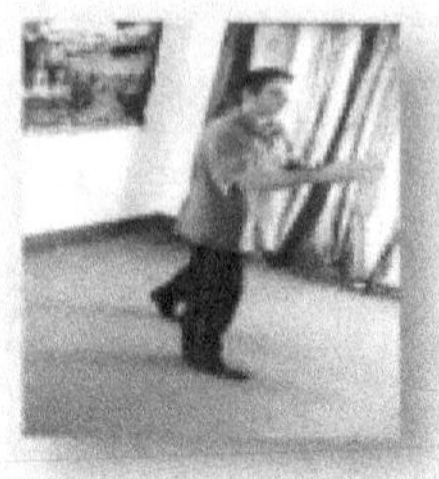 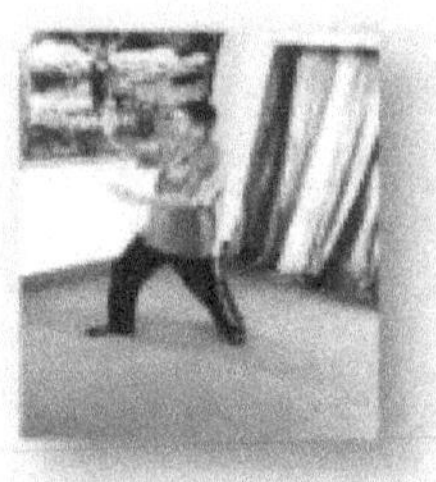

*Transition to the east:* Inhale as the torso and hands turn right to the east direction swivelling on the heels to a balanced stance (a small step with the right foot may be taken). The weight is 70% on the front foot. The left heel lifts off the floor and pauses. The palms are facing each other at chest height, and the fingers of the left hand are pointing at the open palm of the right hand.

*To Southwest:* Exhale as the weight moves back to the left leg, the torso turns right, the right leg lifts and steps to face the southwest corner, heel down first, then flat foot, while the left foot swivels 45 degrees to maintain a balanced stance. Seventy percent of the weight is on the right front foot. Simultaneously, the right palm facing out and away finishes at face height with shoulders relaxed. The left palm is facing out and forward at chest height. Complete the exhale in sync with movements.

# Posture Set Three: Ward Off

## Ward off Left, Right, Bend Bow

Standing in Fair Lady Weaves the Shuttle, facing the southwest corner, the left foot is at the rear 45 degrees outward to maintain a balanced stance. Seventy percent of the weight is on the right front foot. The right palm facing out and away is at face height with shoulders relaxed. The left palm is facing out and forward at chest height.

*Ward off Left: A:* Inhale as the left heel raises off the floor (toes/ball touching floor only) with a slight bend in the knee and 90% weight on the right leg. Simultaneously, the hands turn to hold the 'ball' center at midriff height, the right palm facing down at shoulder height, and the left palm facing up at belly height.

*B:* Exhale as the weight sinks forward in the right front leg, freeing up the left leg to lift and place forward, pointing south, heel down first then flat foot into a balanced stance. Seventy percent of the weight moves onto the left front foot (The torso also faces south).

Simultaneously, the left inward-facing palm is a short distance from the face, while the right palm is inward-facing at the right thigh height. Complete the exhale in sync with the movements.

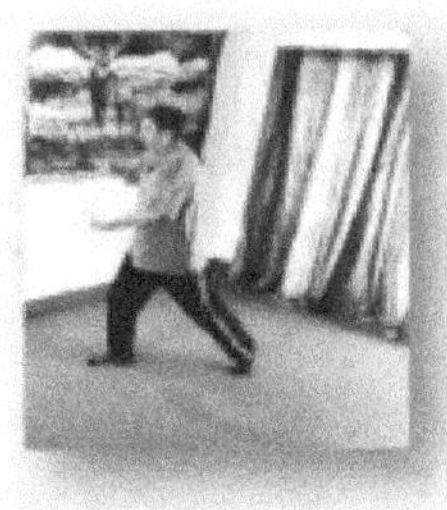 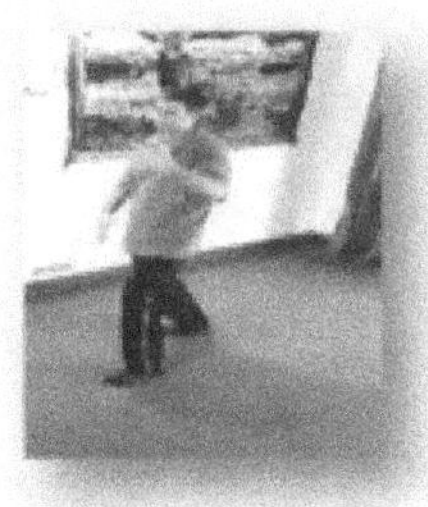 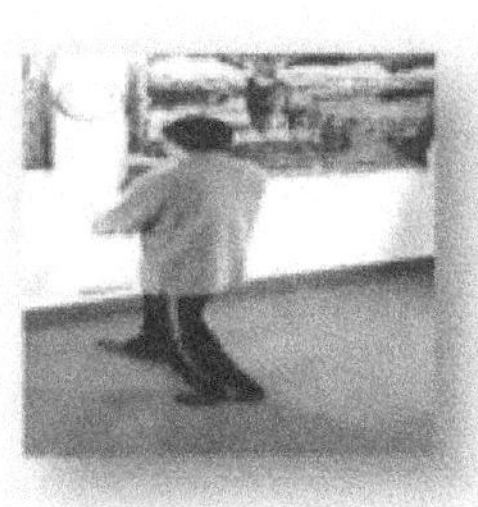

_Ward off Right:_ Inhale as the torso turns to the right, facing west. The body weight sinks into the left leg freeing up the right leg to lift and place, pointing west, heel down first then flat foot into a balanced stance. Seventy percent of the weight moves onto the right front foot, and the hip closes. Simultaneously, the hands turn to hold the 'ball' center at midriff height, the right palm facing down at shoulder height, and the left palm facing up at belly height. Exhale as you settle into the posture.

_Bend Bow:_ Inhale as the hands release the 'ball' separating so that the left hand reaches forward in a light fist at shoulder height while the right hand reaches back in a light fist at shoulder height (imagine bending a bow with an arrow). The feet stay in place. Feel the stretch in the torso. Exhale as you settle into the posture.

# Posture Set Four: Punch Forward

<u>**Punch Forward**</u> (<u>This Punch Forward varies slightly from Punch Forward in Section One</u>)

Standing in Bend Bow, facing west in a balanced stance, with 70% weight on the right front foot - the left hand is reaching forward in a light fist at shoulder height while the right hand is reaching back in a light fist at shoulder height (imagine bending a bow with arrow). The feet stay in place. Feel the stretch in the torso.

*Punch Forward: A:* Inhale as the weight moves back to the left (southwest corner), drawing hands back: the left hand is open, palm facing inwards; the right hand is in a light fist which is held throughout the posture-set. Both hands come to hip height on each frontal side. Simultaneously, with the weight on the left leg, the right foot lifts off and the upper leg raises parallel with the floor into the southwest corner and pauses.

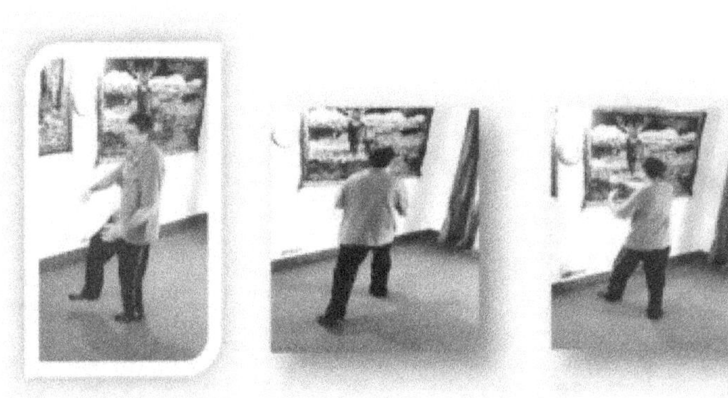

*B:* Exhaling, the whole frame skilfully swivels right to face the northwest corner. The right heel touches down first, then the flat foot. The weight moves forward onto the right leg freeing up the left heel to peel off the floor for a few seconds as one sinks into this posture (appreciate this warrior stance). The hands are at each frontal side of the thigh: the left hand is open, the palm facing inwards; and the right hand is in a fist.

_C:_ Inhaling as the torso, hands, and eyes turn left and the left foot is empty to take a good step to the west, heel touches down first, then flat foot, into a balanced stance. Exhaling, the weight moves westward 70% onto the left leg as the left palm faces inwards at belly height, a short distance from the body, and the right fist punches forward to the west at chest height.

# Posture Set Five: Push and Cross Hands

## *Push and Cross Hands*

Standing in Punch Forward, facing west, in a balanced stance with the weight 70% on the left leg, the left palm faces inwards at belly height, a short distance from the body, and the right fist is extended in a punch forward to the west at chest height.

*Push:* Inhale and lean the body weight back to the rear leg as both hands (palms inward facing) sweep in an arc up the center of the body from hip to shoulder height (imagine drawing up positive energy).

Exhale as the torso and palms at shoulder height push forward and away (as if pushing an object).

Your eyes follow the arc movement as weight settles 70% on the front foot.

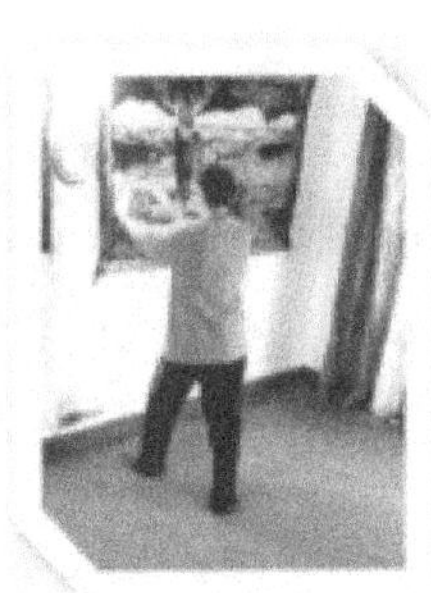
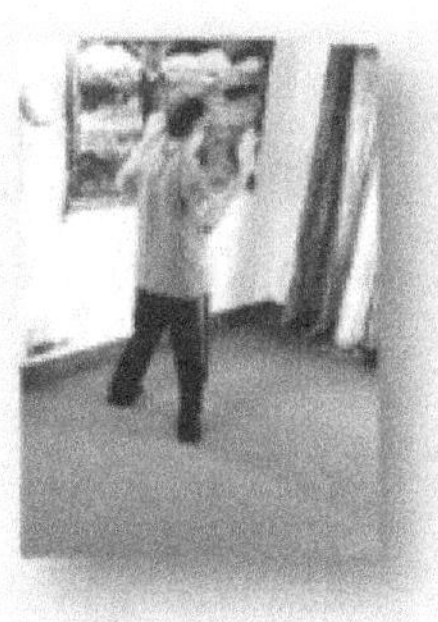
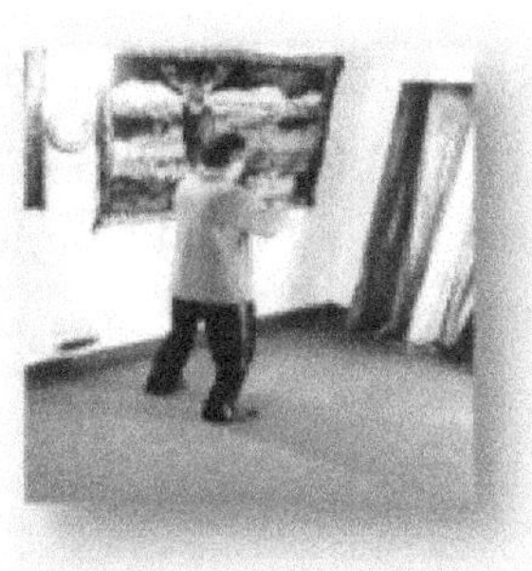

*Cross Hands: A:* Inhale as the torso turns to the right to face north with both hands turning to face north, palms outwards facing at shoulder height. Simultaneously, the left foot swivels on the heel to face north while the right foot stays in place. The elbows can be moved back to effect a shoulder blade squeeze for added measure.

_B:_ Exhale as the right foot is freed up to turn and point north in a parallel stance, weight evenly spread. Simultaneously, both wrists cross in front of the chest, palms inward facing and a short distance from the body.

(Imagine holding a ball of energy – contain the energy that you have cultivated during the form.

Feel the internal. Be aware of the external. Relax the whole frame, suspended from above and rooted to the earth through the feet.

This concludes Section Three and the complete Tai Chi Form. Finish with Moving the Ball to cool down.

## __Moving the Ball__

As one inhales, both hands (palms facing down) float up from the hip away from and in front of the body to shoulder height, and then are slowly drawn toward the body and float back down during the exhale.

This exercise is performed three times in succession. The imagery in this exercise is that from one's center (abdomen region), the hands float up effortlessly as if lifted up by an inflating balloon and then lower as if that balloon is deflating.

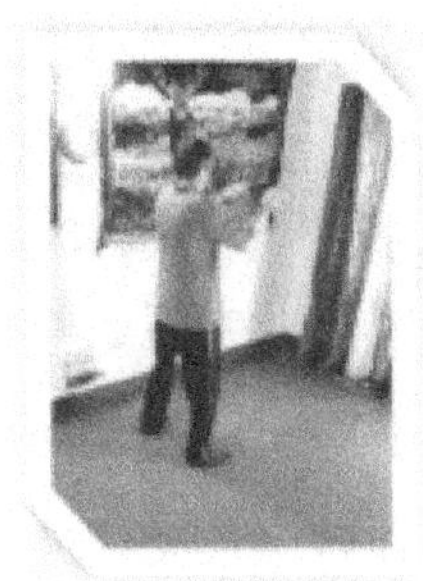 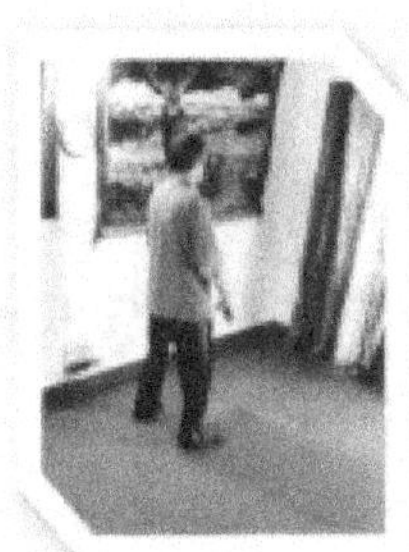 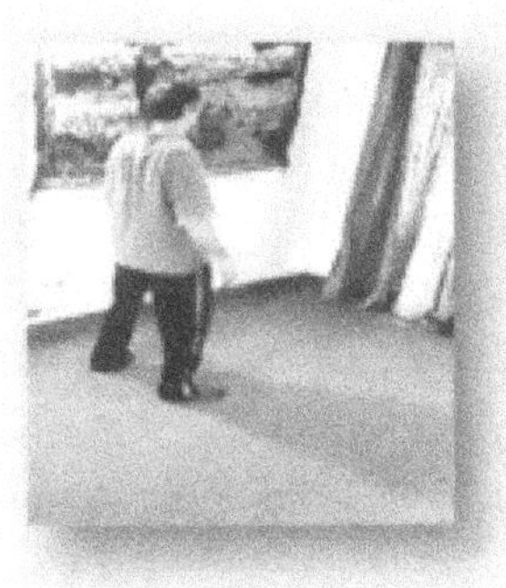

Deep diaphragm breathing is practiced so that during the inhale, air is drawn in to push the diaphragm down expanding the belly and filling the chest; and during the exhale, the belly contracts forcing the air out naturally without any strain. It is good to have a few seconds pause and hold between inhale and exhale movements to increase lung capacity. Traditionally, air is drawn in through the nose and exhaled through either the nose or mouth.

This exercise is performed to begin and end each practice session because it helps to center the practitioner in the here and now; to be present in the moment, still, and aware of the internal and external.

Congratulations on completing all three sections and the Xcelwellness Tai Chi Form. Continue to practice the Tai Chi Form daily to maintain optimum health and well-being.

Xcel Wellness specializes in holistic gentle stretching forms which are popular because they are so effective in gaining results and moving one to an optimum health status.

My wellness books are published under the name Xcel Wellness in online bookstores.

Involved in the Internal Arts since 2005, I am a graduate of Thai Massage, and Natural Therapies and am knowledgeable in Foot Therapy, Gemstones, Numerology, and Nutrition.

I am a certified instructor in Tai Chi and Easy Fitness programs.

**Xcelwellness Tai Chi** takes a holistic approach to health and well-being with each session involving gentle stretching, relaxation, energization, and total body balancing treatments. This 'feel good' therapy enhances one's overall health status for life, work, and play. Xcelwellness Tai Chi can help if you suffer from general poor health, stiffness and fatigue.

Use Xcelwellness Tai Chi to prepare for the workday, to be more focused on activities, to energize, and to sleep more deeply. The comprehensive fitness program with step-by-step guidance for any age group, any place, to fit any lifestyle and schedule.

Xcelwellness Tai Chi can make a big difference for healthy, but very busy people.

**<u>Experience the Xcelwellness Tai Chi Difference</u>**

# Also by J Pilgrim

**The Trionian Saga**
The Trionian Saga - Part One: Beyond the Border Mountains
The Trionian Saga - Part Two: The Hyna Sword
The Trionian Saga - Part Three: The Quest for Lyla


**Standalone**
The Hens in Poultsville
Sleeping with Crystal
Excel Your Wellness: Virtues and Vitamins
The Chi Key: Reflections on You, Me, and the Universe
Body Strengthening Strategy
Xcel Wellness Tai Chi


Watch for more at www.thetrioniansaga.weebly.com.

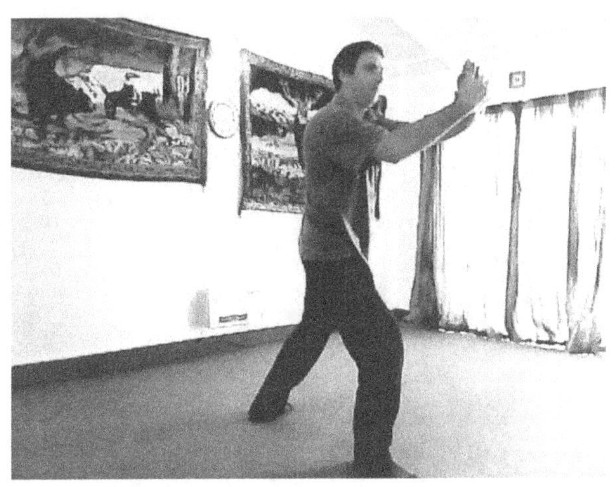

# About the Publisher

**Xcel Wellness has eBooks** published in online bookstores with themes such as wellness, natural therapies, and philosophy.

**Involved in the Internal Arts** since 2004, the author is certified in Thai Massage, Tai Chi, Fitness programs, and Reflexology.

**The author** has eBooks published in all good online stores.

Read more at www.xcelbooks.weebly.com.

www.ingramcontent.com/pod-product-compliance
Lightning Source LLC
Chambersburg PA
CBHW061625130726
47996CB00003B/1126